THE COMPLETE GUIDE TO

LIVING WELL WITH DIABETES

THE COMPLETE GUIDE TO
LIVING WELL WITH DIABETES

Winifred Conkling

A Lynn Sonberg Book

St. Martin's Paperbacks

Notice: This book is intended as a reference volume only, not as a medical manual. The information given here is designed to help you make informed decisions about your health. It is not intended as a substitute for any treatment that may have been prescribed by your doctor. If you suspect that you have a medical problem, we urge you to seek competent medical help.

Mention of specific companies, organizations, or authorities in the book does not imply endorsement by the author or publisher, nor does mention of specific companies, organizations, or authorities imply that they endorse this book, its author, or the publisher.

Internet addresses given in this book were accurate at the time it went to press.

THE COMPLETE GUIDE TO LIVING WELL WITH DIABETES

Copyright © 2009 by Lynn Sonberg Book Associates.

For information address St. Martin's Press, 175 Fifth Avenue, New York, NY 10010.

ISBN: 0-312-94512-4
EAN: 978-0-312-94512-1

Printed in the United States of America

St. Martin's Paperbacks edition / March 2009

St. Martin's Paperbacks are published by St. Martin's Press, 175 Fifth Avenue, New York, NY 10010.

10 9 8 7 6 5 4 3 2 1

For my daughter, Gwendolyn,
diagnosed with type 1 diabetes at age six.

When people ask her, "Will you have diabetes forever?"
she replies, "No, just until there's a cure."

CONTENTS

THE COMPLETE GUIDE TO

LIVING WELL WITH DIABETES

INTRODUCTION

During a family vacation in the summer of 2006, I knew there was something wrong with my six-year-old daughter. She guzzled bottled water and begged for bathroom breaks at least once an hour. At first I blamed the near 100 degree temperatures for her excessive thirst—and the incessant urination. When she put on her bathing suit at the beach, I noticed that she had thinned out since the last day of kindergarten, but I attributed it to a recent growth spurt. By the time we made it home from our week-long trip, I recognized the classic symptoms of diabetes—thirst, frequent urination, and weight loss—and I immediately booked an appointment with the pediatrician.

I had a feeling of impending doom the night before the doctor's visit. I felt certain my daughter had diabetes, and that her life would soon be divided into Before and After Diagnosis. I feared that she had diabetes, but, to be honest, I didn't know much about the disease.

On the morning of the appointment, my daughter skipped breakfast so that the lab could obtain a fasting blood sugar level. In the doctor's office, she surrendered her index finger to the lab technician, who used a lancet to stick her finger and squeeze out a single drop of blood. I held my breath while the glucose meter beeped and processed the data. The number 298 flashed on the display. I didn't need the lab technician or the doctor to tell me what that meant. My daughter had type 1 diabetes.

I couldn't stop tears from streaming down my face while I told my daughter that she had a disease called diabetes. I promised that her father and I would learn everything we needed to know to keep her safe and healthy. I rambled on, offering words of assurance both to comfort her and to convince myself that she would be okay.

A few minutes later, the doctor explained that we needed to go immediately to the hospital where we would stay for three or four days. The pediatric endocrinologist needed to determine her correct insulin dose, and my husband and I needed to learn how to administer insulin, calculate my daughter's carbohydrate demands, and handle dangerous blood sugar highs and lows.

Sitting in the hospital a few hours later, I watched the nurse prepared a syringe with my daughter's first dose of insulin. She looked at me and said, "So, Mom, do you want to do it?"

I am a bit squeamish about needles, but I knew I had no alternative but to step up to the challenge. The nurse explained what to do, and I gave my daughter her first injection of insulin. In that moment—as in many others that followed—I did what I needed to do to take care of my daughter, setting aside my anxieties until I could deal with them later. I always knew I'd do anything within my power to help my children and keep them safe, but I honestly never thought I'd be tested that way.

In the months that followed, I was preoccupied day and night with my daughter's diabetes. She needed to receive insulin and eat a fixed number of carbohydrates at certain intervals throughout the day. She needed to do finger-stick glucose testing at least seven times a day, including at 2 A.M. to make sure her blood sugar levels were neither too high nor too low.

It was an exhausting period of adjustment for all of us, but eventually we developed a more predictable routine. I read everything I could find about diabetes, I met other people with the disease, and I began to relax (a bit).

Diabetes is a fickle and unforgiving disease. It is possible to do everything right, to follow your doctor's orders precisely, and to experience erratic glucose numbers anyway. It took me a while to accept that I didn't have power over this disease. When it comes to diabetes, all you can do is strive to manage the disease, not control it.

Using This Book

While there are many good books on diabetes on the market, this book offers a unique combination of medical information, up-to-date research findings, and practical tips on how to live well with diabetes. In addition to the medical aspects of disease management, the book explores the emotional challenges of living with diabetes. It includes the voices and experiences of many people with type 1, type 2, and gestational diabetes.

The Complete Guide to Living Well with Diabetes is divided into four parts, each covering an important area of care.

Part I provides an overview of how the disease affects the body and how it is diagnosed.

Part II explores approaches to treatment, including the use of insulin and oral medications, as well as the importance of diet and exercise to control blood sugar levels.

Part III outlines common complications of diabetes, both immediate, acute problems and long-term consequences of elevated blood glucose levels.

Part IV covers a range of topics essential to living well with diabetes, including finding a good doctor, managing the emotional stresses associated with the disease, dealing with a diabetic child, and understanding your legal rights. The final chapter offers a brief assessment of future treatments—as well as the possibility of a cure—for type 1 and type 2 diabetes.

A great number of resources are available on the Internet for diabetics. These include Web sites offering basic information, discussion forums, and up-to-the-minute research on related topics. The final pages of the book list some of the leading Web sites of interest to people with diabetes.

Every attempt has been made to ensure the information in this book is as complete and accurate as possible. It cannot, however, replace the advice of your endocrinologist or another medical professional. Use the book as a reference so that you can better understand your diabetes and how to manage it, but specific questions about your treatment plan should be discussed with your health care provider.

PART I

DIAGNOSIS

WHAT IT MEANS TO HAVE DIABETES

CHAPTER 1
OUT OF BALANCE: Understanding Diabetes

When Sarah was a freshman in high school, she didn't feel right. She stopped at the water fountain—and the bathroom—between almost every class. She lost so much weight that the clothes she bought at the beginning of the school year were hanging off of her by December. At first, she assumed her complaints were related to the stress of getting used to high school, but after a couple of months, she worried that something else was wrong.

"I went to the doctor thinking I had mono or some kind of bladder infection that could be cured with antibiotics," said Sarah. "It never occurred to me that I could have type 1 diabetes."

Patrick, on the other hand, made an appointment with his doctor to confirm what he already knew—that he had type 2 diabetes. "Type 2 diabetes runs all through my family," said Patrick, 56. "I never wondered if I would get it, my question was always when."

Patrick had tried to exercise regularly and keep his weight down, but eventually his genetics got the best of him. "For a couple of weeks, I had noticed the symptoms," he said. "I knew what was coming because I had seen other family members go through it." Patrick had learned about the disease from his parents and his older brother—all type 2 diabetics—so he was ready to begin to take responsibility for his disease right away.

For diabetics like Sarah and Patrick, life is a balancing act. People with diabetes—both type 1 and type 2—must carefully watch their blood sugar levels. If their blood sugar levels rise too high and stay there for too long, they risk damage to their nerves and blood vessels, which can cause a number of health problems. But if their blood sugar levels drop too low—even for a few minutes—diabetics can become confused and even lose consciousness.

Sarah has not lost consciousness, but once when her blood sugar was very low, she could no longer take care of herself. "I was swimming with some friends, and we were having such a good time that I lost track of how I was feeling," she said. "When I got out of the pool and sat down, all of a sudden I felt like I couldn't move. My mind was fuzzy but racing at the same time."

One of Sarah's friends realized that something was wrong and gave her juice. "I was scared because I couldn't get the juice for myself," Sarah said. "It's like I forgot what I was supposed to do." Since then, Sarah has been much more careful about testing her blood sugar and eating frequently when she's active.

People without diabetes don't have to worry about making these delicate adjustments in their blood sugar levels. Instead, they have a working pancreas, which regulates the amount of sugar in the bloodstream by releasing the hormone insulin.

Diabetics, on the other hand, must regularly test their blood and adjust their diet and exercise—or their oral medications and insulin injections—to meet the changing conditions. People with diabetes cannot properly convert food into energy, either because their bodies do not produce enough insulin or because their bodies don't properly use the insulin they do produce. When it comes to diabetes, insulin is the hormone that holds the key to stable blood sugar levels.

Understanding the Role of Insulin

Insulin is a hormone produced by the beta cells of the pancreas. Basically, insulin allows sugar to pass into the cells so that it can be used for energy. The process begins when you eat foods containing carbohydrates and your blood sugar level begins to rise. (For a complete discussion of the impact of food on blood sugar, see Chapter 10, Diet.)

In a person without diabetes, this elevated blood sugar level causes the pancreas to release insulin, which, in turn, lowers the blood sugar by allowing the cells to use the sugar. In the body, insulin binds to a receptor on the surface of the cell, which allows sugar to pass through the membrane into the cell. Without the insulin, the sugar can't pass through the cell membrane.

A person with diabetes cannot produce enough insulin to meet the body's demand for it, or the body has become resistant to the insulin produced. Without enough insulin present, the sugar can't pass into the cells, so it builds up in the blood and ultimately passes out in the urine. Because the cells don't have sugar to use in the blood, the body breaks down fat to use for energy. Burning fat releases ketones into the urine, which can be very harmful to the body. (Ketones are discussed in more detail in Chapter 15.)

Before meals and during the overnight hours, the beta cells that produce insulin have a chance to rest. Beta cells continue to produce low levels of insulin to balance the sugar continually produced by the liver, but this is usually a fairly small amount. When you are not eating or digesting the food you have eaten, blood sugar levels tend to be relatively low and stable.

When the system works, the blood sugar is kept in the range of about 70 to 120. After eating, the blood sugar can spike to 200 or more, depending on what food was consumed, but this level typically returns to the normal range within two hours of a meal.

NOTE: In the United States, blood sugar levels are measured in mg/dL or milligrams per deciliter. Many other countries measure blood sugar levels in mM/L or millimoles per liter. (To convert from mM/L to mg/dL, simply multiply by 18.) In this book, blood sugar levels will be stated as numbers without the mg/dL label in most cases.

People with diabetes can have wildly varying blood sugar levels, depending on a number of variables, including the type and amount of food eaten, the amount of insulin taken, exercise, stress, illness, and menstrual cycle (in women), among other factors. For example, a person with diabetes might run high blood sugars for hours after eating a high-fat meal because the fat tends to delay and prolong the rise in blood sugars after the meal. In addition, a person with diabetes who is sick may experience blood sugar levels in the 300s or higher—even without eating—because the body is under stress.

The only way a person with diabetes can overcome these unpredictable fluctuations in blood sugar is to test often and adjust medication as needed. A person is said to have well-controlled diabetes when his or her blood sugar levels stay within the normal range most of the time. That said, even a person with well-controlled diabetes will have average blood sugars higher than a person without diabetes.

YOU ARE NOT ALONE

Diabetes is a growing problem in the United States. Consider the statistics:

- More than 1 million Americans have type 1 diabetes.

- About 17 million Americans have type 2 diabetes.

- About 135,000 pregnant women develop gestational diabetes each year.

- About 16 million Americans have prediabetes, meaning their blood sugar is above normal, but not quite high enough for diagnosis.

A diabetic with poor control tends to have large fluctuations in blood sugar levels. At times, the blood sugar may be well over 300 and at other times it may drop into a dangerously low range. It can be exasperating to attempt to balance volatile blood sugar levels, repeatedly correcting the highs and going too low, then correcting the low and ending up too high.

If you have diabetes, don't expect to maintain perfect control. Keep careful track of your blood sugar numbers and diet over time, and look for patterns. Sometimes conditions change for no apparent reason—it could be a change in the seasons, an undefined stress in your life, or a new brand of breakfast cereal. Be vigilant about monitoring your glucose levels, but don't drive yourself crazy. Just do the best you can, one day at a time, one fingerstick at a time.

The Classic Symptoms

High blood sugar affects the entire body. At the earliest stages, it causes certain common systemic symptoms.

Thirst and Urination: The Diabetic Water Cycle

When your blood sugar is high, your blood becomes thicker. Your brain assumes that your blood is thicker because you are dehydrated, so it sends out a thirst message to encourage you to drink more to thin out your blood. Of course, the excessive drinking leads to excessive urination. Excessive thirst (known as polydipsia) and excessive urination (known as polyuria) don't usually appear until your blood sugar rises above 200 or 250.

Be aware that frequent urination may also be caused

by a urinary tract infection or another medical problem. If you feel the urge to urinate but only eliminate a small amount of urine, this is more likely a symptom of a urinary tract or bladder infection than diabetes. Either way, you need to follow up with your doctor for an appropriate diagnosis and treatment.

Blurred Vision

Diabetes can cause short-term, temporary blurred vision, as well as long-term, permanent problems, such as diabetic retinopathy and blindness (discussed in Chapter 16). Temporary blurred vision happens when the blood sugar is high for several days and the lens, which changes shape to focus your vision, becomes bloated and can't change shape fast enough as you shift your focus from near to far. The lens typically regains elasticity when blood sugar levels return to normal. Generally, vision returns to normal after a couple of days of balanced blood sugar levels, but in some cases it can take up to six weeks for the lens to recover.

Fatigue

People with diabetes often experience fatigue when their blood sugar levels are too high. Without enough insulin, blood sugar levels rise and energy levels drop because the cells are not receiving fuel. The cells are literally starving for the sugar that's building up in the bloodstream.

Fatigue can be mild—hey, who doesn't feel tired once in a while?—or it can be so severe that people can't even drag themselves through the day without a nap. Diabetics taking insulin sometimes feel tired after eating a big meal when the blood sugar level rises before the insulin takes effect.

Weight Loss
Without enough insulin, the sugar level in the blood climbs to a point where it eventually spills out into the urine. A diabetic with poor blood sugar control will lose weight when a significant number of calories are lost in the urine.

If you experience unusual or unexpected weight loss, have your blood sugar checked. It may be in the 300s or 400s, which will cause serious long-term complications in addition to weight loss. Using dangerously high blood sugar levels to lose weight is not safe.

Infections
Infections are common in people with high blood sugar because fungus and bacteria flourish in the high-sugar environment. At the same time the elevated sugar levels compromise the immune system, making it harder for the body to fight off the infection. Common types of infection include yeast infections, urinary tract infections, and gum infections. In addition, high blood sugar can interfere with wound healing, especially wounds on the feet.

Types of Diabetes
There are three types of diabetes:

- Type 1: Most or all of the beta cells in the pancreas fail to produce insulin.

- Type 2: The pancreas produces insulin, but the body does not respond to it.

- Gestational diabetes: The pancreas cannot keep up with the higher demands for insulin when a woman is pregnant.

All three forms of the disease have the same symptoms, but they require different treatments. (The treatments are discussed in Part 2.)

Type 1 Diabetes

Type 1 diabetes is sometimes called insulin-dependent diabetes or juvenile diabetes. The disease lives up to these names because everyone with type 1 diabetes requires insulin and because it usually appears during childhood. Type 1 diabetes can appear in infants or in young adults up to age 30 or older, but most cases are diagnosed in elementary-school-age children.

Sometimes it can be difficult for parents to recognize diabetic symptoms in their young children. Consider four-year-old Andrew, whose mother did not notice the warning signs of diabetes until his preschool teacher pointed out that he was thirsty and used the bathroom more than the other kids his age. The teacher's brother had type 1 diabetes, so she was familiar with the disease and mentioned her concern to Andrew's mother.

"I had assumed that he went to the bathroom so frequently because he was toilet training," Andrew's mother said. "I didn't know anything about diabetes, but I mentioned it to the pediatrician right away. Andrew wasn't overweight, so I didn't think he could have diabetes."

Like Andrew's mother, many people mistakenly believe that people with type 1 diabetes are overweight. In fact, most people who develop type 1 diabetes are average weight or thin. Type 1 diabetes is not linked to obesity and cannot be managed with changes in diet and exercise. That's because in a person with type 1 diabetes, the beta cells in the pancreas have been damaged or destroyed so they can no longer produce insulin. All people with type 1 diabetes depend on insulin injections to remain healthy.

It can be extraordinarily difficult for a person with type 1 diabetes to maintain stable blood sugar levels. Since the pancreas isn't making any insulin, the diabetic must estimate the amount of insulin and carbohydrates required.

Think of your pancreas like a thermostat on your furnace. It turns the furnace off and on many times throughout the day to maintain a reasonably steady temperature. A person with diabetes has a broken thermostat. Instead of a flat temperature, he tends to run hot and cold, with the occasional "just right" in between the extremes. So a diabetic must administer insulin or eat carbohydrates to adjust his blood sugar level throughout the day. Balancing insulin involves educated guesswork, and it won't always result in perfect control.

While every type 1 diabetic has good days and bad days, some people tend to have blood sugar levels that cycle between dangerous highs and dangerous lows several times in a single day. Some doctors call these people with wildly fluctuating blood sugar levels "brittle diabetics." This isn't a separate condition or a type of diabetes; it simply means that a person's diabetes is not under good control. In most cases, blood sugar levels can be stabilized with careful management and consultation with a doctor.

When first diagnosed with type 1 diabetes, many people go through what is known as the "honeymoon period." During this phase, the pancreas continues to produce varying amounts of insulin. Some people maintain stable blood sugar levels and may require very little insulin. Alas, this phase only lasts several months to a year. It may be tempting to imagine that the diagnosis is wrong—you don't have diabetes after all!—but as the months pass and more of the beta cells are destroyed, the disease is fully expressed.

As the parent of a type 1 diabetic, I considered the honeymoon phase a good training period. I had a chance to learn about the disease and become familiar with living with it while my daughter's symptoms were fairly easy to manage.

At first, I was obsessed with trying to figure out how to save her remaining beta cells before the honeymoon ended. I wanted the cells stored so that they could be used at some point in the future when a new treatment is developed (and I sincerely believe it will be). At the time, research was being done on harvested beta cells, but my daughter was not eligible for any of the studies because of her age. Eventually, I had to accept the limitations of medicine at the dawn of the twenty-first century. I reminded myself to feel grateful for the near miraculous treatments that were available. Diabetes care has come a long way just in the last 20 years—and I look forward to what the future will hold.

Within a year of her initial diagnosis, my daughter's

blood sugar numbers began to climb and I frequently had to adjust the amount of insulin she was taking. I knew the honeymoon was over, but by that time I felt more prepared to deal with the challenges of full-blown diabetes.

What Causes Type 1 Diabetes?

Type 1 diabetes is an autoimmune disease. It tends to appear in people with a genetic predisposition to the disease who are then exposed to some kind of environmental trigger, such as viral or bacterial infection. (My daughter had the flu a few months before her diagnosis.) When exposed to a virus or bacteria, the body launches an immune response to search out and destroy the harmful invaders. In a person with type 1 diabetes, the body becomes confused and initiates an autoimmune response, or, more specifically, it mistakenly attacks the beta cells in the pancreas.

People can be genetically susceptible to type 1 diabetes, even if there is no known family history of the disease. (My daughter is the first in our family tree to have type 1 diabetes.) Researchers have identified a number of genes associated with the disease, but having the genes does not guarantee that you will develop the disease. Additional research on this question is ongoing. (For more information on the role of heredity and type 1 diabetes, see Chapter 3.)

Type 2 Diabetes

Type 2 diabetes is sometimes called non-insulin-dependent diabetes or adult-onset diabetes. In this case, the disease is not as aptly named. For one thing, as many as 30 to 40 percent of people with type 2 diabetes eventually do require insulin injections to maintain stable blood sugar levels, although most can control the disease with diet, exercise, and oral medication. In addition, while type 2 diabetes used to occur almost exclusively in people over 40, it now occurs in younger and younger people.

Type 2 diabetes is much more common than type 1. In fact, more than 90 percent of people with diabetes have type 2. It occurs more frequently in overweight people and those who don't exercise. Genes do play a significant role in the development of type 2 diabetes, and it is much more common among Native Americans, Hispanics, and African Americans.

Type 2 diabetes typically develops over a number of years. Most people do not know when the disease first appeared, and some people suffer with symptoms for years before being tested and receiving a diagnosis. Because the onset is typically gradual, some people find excuses to ignore the illness until they develop serious complications.

For example, Trudy suspected that she had diabetes for years before the diagnosis was confirmed by her doctor. She was overweight and inactive, and she didn't want her doctor to tell her she needed to change her lifestyle. "I hate to exercise, so I tried to ignore the disease," the 48-year-old mother of two said. "I avoided the doctor until I developed severe hypertension. I didn't go to the doctor for diabetes, I went because my high blood pressure was giving me headaches."

When her doctor identified the type 2 diabetes in addition to the hypertension, Trudy realized she needed to change her eating and exercise patterns. Two years later, she works out four times a week and has lost about 50 pounds. "I could still lose a few pounds, but I have the problem under control. It's not always easy, but I feel much better than I used to."

Because she changed her lifestyle, Trudy was able to control her diabetes without the use of insulin, although she does take oral diabetes medication. As mentioned earlier, more than one out of every three people with type 2 diabetes ultimately requires insulin to control their blood sugar. This doesn't mean the person has gone from a type 2 to a type 1 diabetic. The type 2 diabetic's pancreas still produces insulin, but that insulin is not sufficient to meet the body's demands. Because the pancreas remains active, most type 2 diabetics who take insulin have an easier time maintaining stable blood sugars than people with type 1 diabetes.

What Causes Type 2 Diabetes?

Genetics plays a significant role in how type 2 diabetes develops, but lifestyle factors are also important. Researchers haven't isolated a single gene responsible for triggering type 2 diabetes, but they have identified several that may contribute to the disease. For example, researchers have located a protein known as PC-1 that appears to set the stage for insulin resistance by shutting down insulin receptors. People with type 2 diabetes tend to have higher levels of this protein than people who do not develop the disease. (For more information on heredity and type 2 diabetes, see Chapter 3.)

In addition to genetics, obesity increases the risk that a person will develop type 2 diabetes. Having too much body fat contributes to insulin resistance, which in turn contributes to type 2 diabetes. The prevalence of type 2 diabetes may also be linked to where body fat is stored. People who store fat in the torso—above the hips—have a higher risk of developing diabetes than those who store fat in their hips and thighs.

Age also may contribute to the risk of developing type 2 diabetes. Half of all cases of type 2 diabetes occur in people over age 55. Since most people tend to gain weight as they age, some researchers question whether older people develop type 2 diabetes more because of their age or their weight.

People who suffer from metabolic syndrome—a constellation of symptoms including high blood sugar, high blood pressure, elevated waist circumference, and low HDL cholesterol—are also at increased risk of developing type 2 diabetes. (Metabolic syndrome is discussed in greater detail in Chapter 2.)

The best way to prevent type 2 diabetes is to exercise regularly and maintain a healthy weight, both steps that help the body use insulin more efficiently. Strategies for changing your lifestyle to minimize your risk of developing diabetes—or to control the disease if you already have it—are discussed in Part 2.

Gestational Diabetes

During pregnancy, hormones produced in the placenta can make a woman resistant to insulin. If a woman's pancreas is overwhelmed by the increased insulin demand during pregnancy, she may develop gestational diabetes, a condition that's similar to type 2 diabetes but only temporary. (A woman with type 1 diabetes who becomes pregnant is not said to have gestational diabetes.)

In most cases, gestational diabetes resolves after the baby is delivered, although women who develop gestational diabetes are at greater risk of developing type 2 diabetes in the future. (Gestational diabetes is discussed in detail in Chapter 13.)

Diabetes with a Known Cause

In some cases, both type 1 and type 2 diabetes can be secondary conditions caused by another medical issue or problem. For example:

- **Drug reactions** can cause elevated blood sugar levels. For example, thiazides (diuretics often used to treat high blood pressure) and steroids (anti-inflammatory drugs) can cause elevated blood sugar levels.

- **Damage to the pancreas,** either from illness or injury, can also cause diabetes. Pancreatitis can damage the pancreas and its ability to produce insulin. Trauma or internal injury can require the removal of the pancreas, causing surgically induced type 1 diabetes.

- **Other diseases,** such as Cushing's syndrome and acromegaly, undermine the effect of insulin, causing diabetes as a side effect.

In situations such as these, the cause of the diabetes is known, although the treatment for the disease is the same as it would be if the exact cause were not known.

While living with diabetes can present significant challenges, the disease itself is fairly straightforward to diagnose using a simple blood test. The following chapter describes the tests that can be used to answer the question: Do you have diabetes?

CHAPTER 2
DIAGNOSIS: Do You Have Diabetes?

Lisa suffered from vaginal yeast infections almost once a month. She felt that as soon as she finished with one round of treatment, the irritating symptoms returned. After almost a year of chronic infections, she went to her doctor for help. The yeast infections weren't the problem, they were a symptom: She had type 2 diabetes. Her high blood sugar levels created a perfect environment for the yeast to thrive.

Sometimes the classic symptoms of diabetes—thirst, frequent urination, weight loss, and chronic vaginal yeast infections—demand attention, prompting a trip to the doctor for a diabetes screening. Other times, the symptoms may be more subtle, allowing the diabetes to go undetected and untreated for long periods of time. In these less obvious cases, diabetes may be discovered with the routine blood work done as part of an annual physical exam. Either way, the diagnosis is made with a simple, almost painless blood test.

Blood Sugar Basics

All blood contains some sugar, which is essential for your body and brain to function normally. If you've ever felt shaky, sweaty, or unable to focus after missing or delaying a meal, you know what it's like to have low blood sugar.

Levels of blood sugar—also known as blood glucose or plasma glucose—fluctuate throughout the day. In a person without diabetes, blood sugar levels may spike after a meal, but the body quickly releases insulin to bring the blood sugar levels back down. Again, a non-diabetic typically has blood sugar levels of about 70 to 120. A person with diabetes has higher—often much, much higher—blood sugar levels.

To diagnose diabetes, a doctor draws a sample of blood to measure your blood sugar levels. If the amount of sugar in the blood is too high, you have diabetes. It's really that simple.

There are three main tests used to diagnose diabetes:

- Fasting blood glucose test: This is a blood glucose test done after overnight fasting. If your fasting blood sugar level is 126 mg/dL or higher, you have diabetes.

- Random blood glucose test: If you experience the classic symptoms of diabetes, your doctor may perform a random (non-fasting) test of your blood sugar. If your blood sugar level is 200 mg/dL or higher in combination with symptoms, you may be diagnosed with diabetes. Random testing of untreated diabetics often shows blood glucose levels in the 300s, 400s, or higher.

- Glucose tolerance test: Your doctor may prescribe an oral glucose tolerance test if the results of the standard tests are borderline or not definitive. The test involves taking a fasting blood glucose sample, followed by drinking a sweet drink containing 75 grams of carbohydrate (sugar). Additional blood samples are taken one, two, and three hours later to determine how well the body can handle the carbohydrate load. Diabetes is diagnosed if the two-hour blood glucose level is 200 mg/dL or higher.

In addition to these diagnostic tests, many obstetricians routinely screen the urine of their pregnant patients for sugar as part of their regular office visits. When blood sugar levels climb above about 200, sugar can spill out into the urine. A urine test wouldn't be used to diagnose gestational diabetes, but it could be used to determine which patients should be sent for an oral glucose tolerance test.

Once a person has been diagnosed with diabetes, many doctors perform blood tests to look for evidence of the antibodies that destroy the pancreas. Antibodies are present in 80 to 90 percent of people with type 1 diabetes at the time of diagnosis. This follow-up test confirms that the person has type 1 diabetes rather than type 2, but the diagnosis of diabetes is not done based on the antibody test alone.

The Gray Zone: At Risk of Developing Diabetes

Some people can dodge the diagnosis of diabetes, but still have blood sugar levels that are higher than desirable. People with blood sugar levels of between 140 and 199 two hours into an oral glucose tolerance test have impaired glucose tolerance (IGT), rather than full-blown diabetes. People with IGT are much more likely to develop diabetes in the future and should make a special effort to exercise, maintain a healthy weight, and have regular physical exams.

Metabolic Syndrome

Metabolic syndrome—sometimes called Syndrome X or insulin resistance syndrome—is a cluster of metabolic risk factors that make a person much more vulnerable to developing type 2 diabetes, as well as cardiovascular disease. Some studies estimate that as many as one out of every four Americans has metabolic syndrome.

Definitions of metabolic syndrome vary, but the American Heart Association defines the condition as three or more of the following:

- High fasting blood sugar: Equal to or greater than 100 mg/dL
- High blood pressure: Equal to or greater than 130/85 or using medication for hypertension
- Elevated waist circumference: Equal to or greater than 40 inches in men or 35 inches in women
- Decreased HDL cholesterol: Lower than 40 mg/dL in men or lower than 50 mg/dL in women
- High triglycerides: Equal to or greater than 150 mg/dL

Most people with metabolic syndrome are older, obese, sedentary, and have some insulin resistance. Researchers debate whether metabolic syndrome is caused by insulin resistance and obesity or whether it is the consequence of these health problems. Some—but not all—people respond to lifestyle changes and can avoid or reverse the syndrome by eating right (limiting sugars and starches) and exercising regularly. Other people require medication to control the various risk factors. Either way, metabolic syndrome should be seen as a warning that you need to take control of your health before you develop serious—and possibly life-threatening—medical problems.

Is Diabetes Forever?

At present, there is no cure for type 1 diabetes. Some people with type 2 diabetes find that they can bring their blood sugar levels back into the normal range without the use of insulin or oral medication by losing weight and exercising regularly. While these efforts are laudable, those who overcome type 2 diabetes should be aware that anyone with a personal history of diabetes is at increased risk of experiencing it again.

The Heart of the Matter

When you first learn that you or someone you love has diabetes, you may feel overcome with emotion. Diabetes is a lifelong, potentially life-threatening disease that can be difficult to manage.

Don't be ashamed to cry or mourn the loss of your old life. It is difficult to accept the diagnosis of a chronic illness that requires a major change in lifestyle. Waves of sadness and anger may come over you for weeks or months after diagnosis, but please remember that the disease can be treated and that breakthroughs in treatment are happening all the time.

Diabetes is a confusing disease, so don't feel you have to become an expert on the condition overnight. There is a lot to learn about the disease, and some of the information can be intimidating and frightening. You owe it to yourself to learn about diabetes, but don't obsess about becoming an expert right away. In the weeks after my daughter was diagnosed, I read almost 20 books about diabetes, but some things I still needed to learn through experience.

Try to find a support group or a community of people who can provide emotional support. Take time to talk about your feelings and ask questions about your illness.

Be aware of depression. Some people find the diagnosis so overwhelming that it takes its toll on their overall outlook on life. If you feel that you may be depressed, seek professional help. (For information on depression and the emotional challenges of living with diabetes, see Chapter 24.)

Some people deny or downplay the importance of the diagnosis, ignoring the disease until it results in serious complications. (The complications of diabetes will be discussed on a topic by topic basis in Part 3.) Even if you don't feel sick, if your blood sugar is high, your body is vulnerable to a wide range of possible neurological and circulatory problems.

Of course, it is possible to live a full and healthy life with diabetes, but you will need to make a special effort to take good care of yourself. You will face some challenges that non-diabetics do not have to face, but most of these can be managed with effort. You can survive and thrive with diabetes, and one of the most important steps you can take is to learn all you can about the disease.

In addition to managing their own health, many people with diabetes worry about the risk of their children also developing the disease. The following chapter discusses the genetic risk of passing diabetes on to your children.

CHAPTER 3
THE GENETIC LINK

Kimberly thought she knew a lot about living with type 1 diabetes: She grew up with a brother and sister who were both diagnosed with the disease before their eighth birthdays. She now knows even more: Both of her elementary-school-aged children also have the disease.

While some people, such as Kimberly, have a strong family history of diabetes, many others do not. Eric can trace his family tree back to the Revolutionary War, and he has no history of the disease. "I'm not sure why, but I'm the first one in my family to get diabetes," said the 23-year-old who was diagnosed with type 1 diabetes at age 17. "It caught us all by surprise."

When people learn that they have diabetes, many look at their family history and either feel that they were destined to develop the disease because other family members have had it—or, like Eric, they may feel caught off guard because they're the first in the family to be diagnosed.

Diabetes is not inherited in a simple pattern. Researchers know that genetics plays some role in determining who gets the disease, but there are a number of other factors that come into play as well. Specifically, researchers believe that something in the environment triggers diabetes among people who are genetically susceptible to the disease.

At this point, scientists have isolated several genes that make people more vulnerable to diabetes, but there is a great deal about the genetics of diabetes that remains a mystery. For example, most Caucasians who develop type 1 diabetes have genes called HLA-DR3 or HLA-DR4. Less research has been done on other ethnic groups, but HLA-DR7 may affect African Americans, and HLA-DR9 may put the Japanese at risk. People who inherit these genes are more vulnerable to diabetes, but the genes alone will not cause the disease; these genes must be turned on or activated by an environmental stressor, such as exposure to a virus or bacteria.

Unfortunately, there's a long way between knowing you're at risk and being able to do anything about it. In the future, researchers may be able to look at a map of a person's genes and determine if that person is likely to develop diabetes and then take steps to prevent the disease from being expressed, but we're not there yet.

Heredity and Type 1 Diabetes

In most cases of type 1 diabetes, people with the disease inherit risk factors from both parents. The genetically susceptible person must then be exposed to something in their environment that triggers the disease. If the genes for type 1 diabetes aren't activated, a person may live a long and healthy life without ever developing the disease. In other words, it takes both a genetic predisposition and an environmental trigger to cause diabetes.

Researchers have studied identical twins to assess the role of heredity in type 1 diabetes. Evidence suggests that genes play some role, but genes alone don't tell the whole story. If type 1 diabetes were strictly genetic, if one identical twin developed the disease, the other one would as well because they have the same genetic makeup. What researchers found is that if one identical twin had type 1 diabetes, the other twin developed the disease about 35 percent of the time. This indicates that genetics is one factor but that something else is at work, too.

That's where the environmental trigger comes in. Unfortunately, no one knows exactly what factor or factors may set off the immune response. Viral or bacterial exposures may play a role, but no particular exposure is common to all people with type 1 diabetes. Toxins in the air, water, or diet may also be a factor, but, again, researchers have not been able to isolate any toxic exposure experienced by all people with type 1 diabetes.

A laboratory blood test known as the islet cell antibody test can be used to prove that the beta cells in the pancreas are being destroyed by an autoimmune response. This test can yield positive results—meaning there is evidence that beta cells are being destroyed—several years before the symptoms of type 1 diabetes first appear. This indicates that the disease may be present for an extended period of time, not just the weeks or months before diagnosis. A virus or bacterial infection may stress the body and bring out the symptoms of the diabetes for the first time, but the disease may have been damaging the body behind the scenes for some time.

Are Your Other Children at Risk?

Sometimes parents of children with type 1 diabetes want to have the other children in the family tested to see if they have antibodies present indicating that they may be vulnerable to developing diabetes in the future. Many doctors discourage parents from doing this test because at this time there is nothing that can be done to prevent the disease from developing. In addition, some people may be vulnerable to the disease but never develop it for reasons that are not well understood. In addition to my daughter with type 1 diabetes, I have two other children, and my husband and I have not had them tested for anti-

---

WHAT IS YOUR RISK OF DEVELOPING TYPE 1 DIABETES?

Less than 0.2% . . .
. . . for the population at large. (The risk is lower among African Americans and higher among Scandinavians.)

Less than 1% . . .
. . . if a grandparent or cousin had type 1 diabetes.

Less than 2–3% . . .
. . . if your mother had type 1 diabetes. (The risk is at the higher end of the range if your mother developed diabetes before age 11.)

---

bodies suggesting diabetes. If either of them develops diabetes at some future date, I will do everything in my power to help them, but at this point, I've got enough on my plate without borrowing trouble.

Heredity and Type 2 Diabetes

Much of what we know about the genetics of type 2 diabetes comes from research on high-risk populations, such as certain Indian tribes where as many as 80 percent of people over 55 develop the disease. In addition, studies of twins with type 2 diabetes have found that if one identical twin has type 2 diabetes, there is at least a

---

Less than 6% . . .
. . . if your father had type 1 diabetes. (The risk is at the higher end of the range if your father developed diabetes before age 11.)

About 3–10% . . .
. . . if one sibling has type 1 diabetes.

About 35–50% . . .
. . . if your identical twin has type 1 diabetes.
Frankly, these odds aren't too bad, which may help to explain why some people feel that type 1 diabetes came out of nowhere since there were no known family members with the disease. Other family members may have had the genetic predisposition but not the environmental trigger to activate those genes.

---

90 percent chance that the other twin will develop the disease as well.

Lifestyle—or, more specifically, obesity—also plays a significant role in the development of type 2 diabetes. People who are overweight tend to be insulin resistant, meaning that a unit of insulin lowers their blood sugar less than it does in a person who is not insulin resistant. For this reason, the pancreas of an overweight person must put out proportionately more insulin to maintain healthy blood sugar levels. If the pancreas can't keep up with the increased demand, then the person develops type 2 diabetes. Fortunately, weight loss can often reverse the condition by easing the demands on the pancreas.

WHAT IS YOUR RISK OF DEVELOPING TYPE 2 DIABETES?

Less than 6% : . . .
. . . for the population at large. (The rate is higher among Native Americans, African Americans, and Hispanics.)

About 4–7% . . .
. . . if your mother or father has type 2 diabetes.

About 12% . . .
. . . if both your mother and father have type 2 diabetes.

If you have already been diagnosed with diabetes, your current challenge is to learn how to live with the disease on a day-to-day basis. The next section of the book looks at treatments for both type 1 and type 2 diabetes. The next chapter examines the goals of your treatment. You need to understand the targets you're setting for yourself so that you can measure your progress and keep your diabetes in check.

About 13% . . .
. . . if one sibling has type 2 diabetes.

As much as 90% . . .
. . . if an identical twin has type 2 diabetes.

These odds are somewhat less reliable than the odds for type 1 diabetes since they depend on other risk factors, such as weight and exercise patterns. If you're in a higher-risk category, you can lower your odds by maintaining a healthy weight and exercising regularly—two habits that will not only lower your risk of developing type 2 diabetes but will offer many other health benefits as well.

PART II

TREATMENT

WHAT YOU NEED TO DO TO CONTROL YOUR DIABETES

CHAPTER 4
SETTING GOALS: What Your Blood Sugar Should Be

When she was first diagnosed with type 2 diabetes, Diane felt nervous every time she tested her blood sugar. She wasn't afraid of the finger-stick, she was afraid of the results. "In the beginning, my heart pounded every time I tested," said Diane, 52. "I didn't know what to expect. One time I'd be 72 and the next time I'd be 142. I wanted my numbers to be consistent, but they never were."

After a couple of weeks, Diane realized that while her numbers fluctuated, they were usually within her target range. She was doing a good job of controlling her diabetes after all, and when she got an unusually high or low reading, she was often able to figure out how her food intake may have changed her blood sugar level.

As was the case with Diane, your blood sugar changes from moment to moment throughout the day, based on a wide range of factors. Of course, food and insulin—whether from your pancreas or from an injection—make a huge difference in your blood sugar, but exercise, emotional excitement, sleep patterns, hormone levels, stress, illness, and other factors also affect your numbers.

As you watch your blood sugar levels bounce up and

down, you can probably recognize certain patterns and anticipate basic trends, but there are times when your blood sugar seems completely unpredictable. When that happens—and it will—try to analyze what's going on in your life and make the necessary adjustments to your diabetic routine.

I learned early on that every time my daughter eats pizza or another high-fat food, she tends to go low after eating; then her blood sugar skyrockets four to six hours after finishing the meal. Why? Because the fat slows the absorption of the carbohydrate in the digestive system, so she gets too much insulin at first and not enough hours later when her blood sugar is still climbing. (This problem has been solved with her insulin pump, which allows her to take some insulin with her meal and to spread the rest out over an extended period.)

Other times, particularly after breakfast, her numbers can shoot up over 300 before her morning insulin kicks in enough to bring her blood sugar back into balance. (We try to give her insulin before eating, but she still has a fairly significant rise in morning blood sugar.)

I know I want to prevent these uncomfortable spikes in blood sugar, but it's not easy. As I've learned the hard way, it's one thing to set goals, and quite another thing to achieve them. Sometimes it feels that the more closely I try to control my daughter's blood sugar, the more unpredictable her numbers become. If you're like me, you may find it difficult to accept that you can follow all the rules of good diabetes management and still have less than perfect results. Alas, you must aim for appropriate target numbers; do your best to achieve those goals, and then accept that more often than you'd like you will fall short of your goal. Forget perfection; settle for reasonably close to your target.

Defining Normal

For a person without diabetes, a fasting blood sugar level is usually under 100 in the morning, although that number typically bounces around between 70 and 120 throughout the day. After eating a meal containing carbohydrates, a healthy person's blood sugar rises to 120 or 130, but not usually above 140. (It can go higher, of course, depending on the amount and type of carbohydrates eaten.) Within two to four hours of eating, the blood sugar drifts down again, back into the 70 to 120 baseline range. All day, the blood sugar levels rise and fall, with peaks and valleys that look like rolling hills.

For a person with type 1 diabetes, those rolling hills tend to turn into alpine mountains, with sharp points and steep inclines and declines. The peaks are higher and the changes are more abrupt. That's because your body makes quick turns and adjustments when injected insulin takes effect. People with type 2 diabetes tend to fall somewhere in between, depending on the medication they take and how careful they are with their diet and exercise.

Don't make yourself crazy by setting unrealistic goals. If you have diabetes, your blood sugar profile won't look like the profile of a person without diabetes. You will have highs and lows, but you can go a long way toward smoothing out those peaks and valleys by eating right and taking your medication.

You will need to talk with your doctor about setting your personal blood sugar targets. Everyone is different and every doctor has different expectations, based on a person's age, activity level, and lifestyle. As a basic goal, you probably want to keep your average blood sugar level below 150 to minimize your risk of long-term complications.

For an adult with diabetes, tight control means keeping blood sugars as close to normal levels as possible. Poor control means running high much of the time. "Lability" or "brittleness" are terms that refer to blood sugar levels that fluctuate wildly, even if the average numbers are okay.

THE DAWN PHENOMENON

In the early morning—between 4 A.M. and 8 A.M.— your body releases growth hormones, which provide a sort of wake-up call to your body. These hormones depress the effectiveness of insulin, causing a rise in blood sugar so that you'll have plenty of energy to get you moving for the day. This pattern has been called the Dawn Phenomenon.

If you have diabetes, this boost in blood sugar can push your blood sugar into unhealthy levels. If you tend to wake up with high blood sugar, consider testing at midnight and then again at 4 A.M. If your blood sugar is normal at midnight and rises until morning, then you may need more insulin during the overnight hours. Talk to your doctor about ways to adjust your insulin dose.

Children with diabetes often have wider blood sugar target ranges. When my daughter was first diagnosed with type 1, her endocrinologist recommended that she keep her blood sugar between 80 and 180. Now that she's on a pump, her target range is 80 to 160. Children often have higher ranges of acceptable blood sugar levels because they tend to be active and have very volatile blood sugar numbers. I know my daughter's blood sugar can drop 100 points in 15 or 20 minutes if she's running around outside. In addition, young children often have undetected low blood sugar levels because they are unable to tell someone they feel symptoms of a low.

A1c Testing

Researchers believe that blood sugar averages determine your long-term risk of diabetic complications, not the occasional highs and lows. To assess average blood sugar levels, doctors use the hemoglobin A1c (glycohemoglobin) test, which measures the amount of sugar coating your red blood cells. This blood test gives you an excellent idea of how well you have controlled your blood sugar over the past two to three months. (A1c testing is described in greater detail in the following chapter.)

Some people can become obsessive about maintaining low A1c numbers, even at the risk of experiencing dangerous lows. Ken prided himself on his tight control and A1c numbers that were within the range of people without diabetes. When he began experiencing regular bouts of low blood sugar, his doctor suggested that he allow his blood sugars to run a little bit higher. He found it very difficult to honor his advice, although he appreciated the serious risk of low blood sugar episodes.

"For years I had worked to keep my A1c numbers down," said Ken, 59. "It was hard for me to let my blood sugar run a little bit higher. I had a couple of fairly serious lows, so I knew what the doctor was telling me made sense."

As you might expect, people with type 1 diabetes tend to have somewhat higher A1c goals compared to people with type 2 diabetes. As noted earlier, it's much harder for someone with type 1 diabetes to maintain stable blood sugar levels, so it is also harder for them to obtain low A1c results.

Your individual goals may change over time. You might need to tighten your goals if you note that you are experiencing periods of high blood sugar, if you are considering pregnancy, or if you develop complications related to your diabetes. On the other hand, you may want to relax your goals and allow your blood sugar to run a little higher if you are experiencing unexpected lows, if you're dealing with another health problem or planning an important event (such as a business meeting or a long drive) and you don't want to go low.

If you receive disappointing A1c results, don't beat yourself up about how you've failed to stick to your diet, exercise plan, or testing routine. You can't change the past. Try to identify the obstacles that prevented you from reaching your goals in the last few months and address them. Take it one day at a time and ask your healthcare provider for suggestions on how to adjust your medication or insulin dosing or how to change your meal plan to reach your goals. Everyone goes through periods in which it becomes more difficult to control their diabetes. Just start again and resolve to do your best.

While it's important to set goals, you will need to test your blood sugar regularly to find out how well you are achieving your goals. The following chapter discusses glucose monitoring and A1c testing—the two most important tools you can use to test your blood sugar levels.

CHAPTER 5

GLUCOSE MONITORING: Testing Your Sugar Levels

Patty suspected she had type 2 diabetes for years before she discussed the matter with her doctor. She wasn't concerned about changing her diet or starting an exercise plan, but she was morbidly afraid of testing her blood sugar several times a day. When her doctor confirmed her suspicions at an annual physical, she burst into tears and confessed her fear of needles and blood. Her doctor referred her to a diabetes educator, who helped her learn to control her anxiety about testing.

While most people with diabetes aren't as worried about testing as Patty, they often grow tired of the finger-sticks required for regular blood sugar testing. Unfortunately, monitoring your blood sugar several times a day at a minimum is an essential part of caring for your diabetes.

Yes, you may feel thirsty, tired, and the need to urinate a lot when you're high—or shaky, sweaty, and confused when you're low—but these symptoms don't usually appear until your blood sugar is way out of the target zone—over 200 or below 60.

In addition, your body's warning signs don't always

work. If your blood sugar is high for a few days, you will get used to feeling high and you will become less aware of the symptoms. When your blood sugar drops, you may feel low even when it is a healthy 90 or 100, because your body had become acclimated to the higher level. This problem corrects itself once your blood sugar is under control, but it shows that you cannot rely on your symptoms to provide foolproof feedback. Bottom line: The only reliable way to find out whether your blood sugar is high, low, or in the target zone is to test.

Using a Blood Glucose Meter

You can monitor your blood sugar level at home with a handheld blood sugar meter or glucometer. It's easy to test your blood sugar, no matter what brand meter you use:

1. Wash and dry your hands. Any sugar or traces of food on your hands can give you a false high reading.

2. Wipe your finger with an alcohol swab and let it dry. If it isn't dry, you'll dilute the blood and get a bad reading.

3. Choose a spot on the side of one of your fingers. Avoid the tip of your finger where there are more nerve endings.

4. Using a lancet, a spring-loaded device with a retractable sharp blade, poke your finger and squeeze out a drop of blood. Most lancets can be

adjusted so that you don't need to poke yourself any deeper than necessary. (I am partial to lancets in preloaded drums, rather than the style that requires handling individual exposed blades each time you test. They're easy to use and you won't accidentally cut yourself.)

5. Touch the drop of blood with the test strip. Within 30 seconds or so, the meter will flash your blood sugar number.

While each system is different, most meters use test strips that contain an enzyme—either glucose oxidase or hexokinase—that reacts with the drop of blood. The system either measures the color of the strip (the darker the color, the higher the blood sugar), or it measures an electrical current.

Most systems must be kept calibrated, meaning that each time you open a new container of test strips, you need to check the meter for accuracy. To do this, you will use a control solution provided by the manufacturer instead of a drop of blood in your meter. The test results should be within a range established by the meter manufacturer. (If you test and your meter is out of the correct range, you can call the customer service number for help or a replacement meter.)

Almost everyone with diabetes gets used to the finger pricks. My daughter only complains on the days that her numbers are erratic and she has to test as many as ten times a day (and the times I have to wake her up to test in the middle of the night). Even if you're anxious about the finger-sticks at first, you'll become familiar with the routine, and testing will become one more thing you do during the course of your day.

If you have trouble squeezing out a drop of blood from your finger, try washing your hands with warm water and wiggling your fingers to increase circulation before you test. If you can't scare up a drop of blood, try swinging your arms in wide circles to allow centrifugal force to help. You may also need to adjust the lancet to stick a little bit deeper next time.

Most meters provide readings within 10 percent of the actual blood sugar. In other words, if your blood sugar is 100, the meter should read anywhere from 90 to 110. Meters become less accurate at the extremes—over 400 or less than 50.

If you get an unexpected reading, wipe your finger thoroughly and test again. You should also keep a backup meter with you in the house and when you're traveling on vacation or business. Also make sure you keep extra batteries on hand so you don't have to run to the drug store in the middle of the night if your meter's battery fades out.

Do not share your meter or testing supplies with anyone else. Hepatitis, AIDS, and other blood-borne viruses can be spread from blood-to-blood contact, and accidents can happen. Keep your medical supplies to yourself.

Continuous Glucose Monitors

Several companies have developed systems to continuously track blood sugar levels, and new products are in development. With these devices, a sensor is inserted under the skin, where it stays for three to five days, depending on the company.

These system's have a transmitter and a receiver. The transmitter contains a battery, an electronic sensor, and a radio transmitter. (My daughter's device is about the size of a quarter.) The sensor is placed under the skin, into the subcutaneous layer of fat. The transmitter sends a radio signal to the pump, which then translates the radio signal into a blood sugar reading.

Continuous glucose monitors provide ongoing blood sugar readings, however, there is a lag time—about 5 to 10 minutes—between the glucose level in the blood and the level in the subcutaneous fat layer. For this reason, you should always test your blood sugar with a finger-stick before taking insulin.

We bought a continuous glucose monitor for my daughter as soon as they were made available for children. In my experience, the monitors are especially helpful at showing trends. At a glance, I can see if her blood sugar level is climbing, falling, or staying flat. This helps me put her number in context and make judgments about what treatment she might need.

In addition, the monitors can be set with high and low alarms. These warnings provide welcome reminders to test and make adjustments by either adding insulin or carbs to bring the blood sugar back into the target zone.

Frankly, I have become dependent on the monitor. I feel much more comfortable allowing my daughter to go outside and play—as well as to experiment with foods she enjoys (even if I'm not confident about the carb count)—because I can see how her body is adjusting to the changing circumstances. Without stopping for a finger-stick, I can get a general idea of how well controlled her blood sugar is at any given point in time. I also rest easier at night and when she is at school because I know that she will hear an alarm if her blood sugar falls too far out of her target range.

How Often to Test

Self-monitoring blood sugar is the foundation of good blood sugar control. You need to follow your doctor's recommendations, but most people use these guidelines:

- Whether you have type 1 or type 2 diabetes, test your blood sugar level whenever you feel high or low. The only way you can know your blood sugar is to test.

- If you have type 1 diabetes, you should test before breakfast, lunch, dinner, and bedtime—and any other time you eat or need to take additional insulin. Many people also test between 2 and 3 A.M.

- If you have stable type 2 diabetes and your blood sugar levels tend to be in the normal range, you need to test several times a day to make sure your blood sugar levels remain normal. If you are taking insulin, you need to test three or four times a day; vary the times you test. If you are taking oral diabetes medications, test in the morning and at least one additional time during the day.

- If you are changing your medication, you need to test frequently to assess how your body is responding to the change in your treatment plan.

- If you have a continuous glucose monitor, you will need to test with a finger-stick before administering insulin.

Blood sugar monitors have revolutionized the care of diabetes, allowing people to have much tighter control of their diabetes. The machines are becoming smaller and they require less blood than ever before.

Keeping Records

You're going to need to keep a log of your various blood sugar readings, as well as other important information about your diabetes. Your doctor will give you a log book or a sample page to copy to record your data. (Most doctors have their own preferred format.)

My daughter's doctor gave us a form, but I found that some of the boxes were so small I couldn't make all the necessary notes. Instead of relying exclusively on the forms, I jot down the information in a composition book, then copy the data onto the doctor's sheet. This may sound like more work, but it helps me keep track of special circumstances (holidays, illnesses, travel, school events) that may have affected her blood sugar on a particular day.

By recording the blood sugar readings in a log, you will recognize patterns that will help you make necessary adjustments in medication (both insulin and oral medications). You may also see patterns in blood sugar in response to certain foods you eat or activities you do. As you become proficient at identifying patterns, you will learn how to anticipate certain blood sugar changes and treat them before your blood sugar runs high or low.

It may take several weeks to fine-tune your diabetes routine—and then you will need to make continual adjustments. Don't change the treatment when your blood sugar levels are bouncing around, but do make adjustments in your routine when you recognize a pattern in your blood sugar three times a week or more. For example, if you find that your blood sugar is too high in the mid-afternoon three or more times a week, you may need to take more insulin to cover the food you eat at lunch.

At first, you will need to discuss the matter with your doctor before making any insulin adjustments. Over time, you will get a feel for the relationship between your medication, food, activity level, and blood sugar level, and you will be able to make minor adjustments on your own.

If you look at your log book and see that your numbers are erratic, but you aren't sure how to make a correction, ask your doctor for help. (Don't ignore the problem until the next time you see your doctor.) You can expect to make adjustments on an ongoing basis.

It can be especially difficult to keep children with diabetes under good control because they are constantly growing and their activity levels vary widely. Don't expect a child's insulin dosages to remain stable very long. Dealing with diabetes requires a one-day-at-a-time approach.

A1c Testing

Hemoglobin A1c is a test used to measure average blood sugar levels over an 8- to 12-week period. (Glycated hemoglobin and glycohemoglobin refer to similar tests that also assess blood sugar control.)

Hemoglobin is a protein inside the red blood cells that

carries oxygen from the lungs to the cells. When exposed to sugar, hemoglobin becomes glycated (joined with the glucose molecules). Once glycated, the hemoglobin holds on to that sugar coating during its entire four-month life span. The higher the blood sugar, the greater the amount of sugar stuck to the outside of the hemoglobin.

The A1c test measures the amount of glycohemoglobin in your red blood cells. By measuring the glucose stuck to the red cells, researchers can determine the average blood sugar since that cell has been in circulation. The A1c doesn't provide any information about current blood sugar levels, but it does give you a good idea of how well you have been able to control your blood sugar during the past three or four months. It's sort of a report card on how well you've controlled your diabetes. Most doctors recommend A1c testing four times a year.

Most laboratories consider normal A1c levels for a non-diabetic person to be 6.4 percent or lower. The following table gives you a general idea of average blood sugars based on A1c results.

A1c (%)	Average Blood Sugar Level
6	135 MG/DL
7	170
8	205
9	240
10	275
11	310
12	345
13	380

While A1c gives an excellent assessment of average blood sugar, it doesn't indicate how variable the blood sugar has been. Your diabetes may be out of control—extreme highs and lows—but your average blood sugar may appear okay. Wildly fluctuating blood sugar levels do not indicate good diabetic control, even if your A1c results are reasonable. You need to strive for balanced blood sugars with low A1c results.

Another test known as fructosamine is similar to the A1c test, but it provides average blood sugar levels over a two-week period. This test is often used to monitor blood sugar control during pregnancy, when it's important to keep tighter control of blood sugar levels.

Urine Glucose Testing

As mentioned earlier, sugar spills out into the urine when your blood sugar level reaches about 180 or 200. Reagent sticks can be dipped into the urine to measure glucosuria, or sugar in the urine. The tip of the stick contains an enzyme that reacts with the sugar; the darker the stick becomes, the greater the amount of sugar in the urine.

A generation ago, before personal glucose monitoring devices were available, urine test strips were the primary tool for monitoring blood sugar levels. Many people with diabetes routinely spilled low levels of sugar to avoid lows.

Urine testing is crude and often inaccurate. Blood sugar levels change rapidly, and urine sugar levels are at a minimum several hours out of date. Something as simple as drinking water can dilute the urine and alter the blood sugar results. In addition, urine testing shows if your blood sugar has been high, but it can't detect a blood sugar low. This is not an effective way to assess blood sugar levels.

So what is the purpose of urine testing? Some obstetricians routinely screen their pregnant patients' urine for sugar as a simple way of detecting gestational diabetes, which can show up at any point in a pregnancy. When used for this purpose, it can be a useful tool, but urine testing is not a part of regular diabetes care.

Urine Ketone Testing

Ketones in the urine indicate the breakdown of fat in the body. When the body doesn't have access to food for a period of 12 to 16 hours, it may turn to stored fat for fuel. When the body burns fat, ketones may appear in the urine. If a diabetic doesn't have enough insulin, ketones may appear in the urine; this can easily become a medical emergency known as ketoacidosis. (For more information on ketoacidosis, see Chapter 15.)

For a person with diabetes, urine ketone testing is an important way of assessing whether the body is approaching ketoacidosis when blood sugar levels run high. A reagent stick is placed in the urine and the pad on the end of the stick changes color; the darker the color, the higher the level of ketones. Moderate or large amounts of ketones in the urine indicate a medical emergency; contact your doctor immediately.

It is possible to develop ketoacidosis with blood sugars in the 200s, so don't assume you need to test for ketones only if your blood sugar is severely elevated. Keep urine ketone test strips on hand, and test for ketones if your blood sugar remains high for several consecutive tests or if you are sick.

If you are responsible about monitoring your blood sugar levels, you will probably detect many episodes of low blood sugar—hypoglycemia—before they become dangerous. The following chapter discusses the problem of low blood sugar and how you can recognize and treat symptoms as soon as possible.

CHAPTER 6
TOO LOW: Hypoglycemia

On a lovely spring day, my daughter and her classmates raced around the playground at school collecting acorns and putting them in paper bags. After about a half hour, the students lined up to return to the classroom. When she wasn't distracted with all of the activity, my daughter realized that she didn't feel right. She went to the clinic and got tested. Her blood sugar was 25. She immediately drank two juice boxes, and within a few minutes she was fine—but I still feel haunted by my fears of what could have been.

Other people with diabetes also experience dangerous blood sugar lows. Todd had adjusted his medication for type 2 diabetes, but he didn't want to set the alarm to test his blood sugar in the middle of the night. In the morning, his daughter could barely rouse him. She gave him orange juice and he recovered within a few minutes. "I don't know how low I went," Todd said. "I now test in the night any time there's a change in my routine."

Diabetics can expect to experience episodes of low blood sugar, or hypoglycemia, on occasion. These episodes can be frightening and dangerous, but most severe cases can be prevented with vigilant care.

Technically, hypoglycemia is defined as a blood sugar level below 60, but people experience clinical symptoms of hypoglycemia at differing blood sugar levels. Most people with diabetes refer to these experiences of low blood sugar as "insulin reactions," "hypos," or "lows." Hypoglycemia is dangerous, and, unfortunately, it is the most common complication for people taking insulin. By some estimates, people who take insulin experience lows an average of once a week, although most of these lows are not severe. Hypoglycemia can also occur in people taking medication for type 2 diabetes.

Most people with diabetes develop mild hypoglycemia that is quickly corrected with intake of carbohydrates. In severe cases, hypoglycemia causes seizures, coma, or even death. With a blood sugar reading of 25, my daughter was at serious risk of losing consciousness. When I recounted the experience to her doctor, she casually said, "Well, I'm surprised she didn't have a seizure."

When my daughter goes low, she looks pale and clammy, her hands tremble, and she gets spacey. She once went low when the family went out to dinner, and we knew something was wrong because she made foolish mistakes while playing tic-tac-toe. This time when we tested her blood sugar, the reading was 37.

Hypoglycemia affects everyone differently. Symptoms can come and go quickly, so anyone with diabetes should become familiar with their patterns so that they can treat hypoglycemia before the condition becomes dangerous.

The most common symptoms include:

Physical
- Shaking or trembling
- Sweating
- Rapid heartbeat
- Nervousness
- Dizziness or light-headedness
- Poor coordination
- Hunger
- Fatigue

Mental
- Headache
- Difficulty concentrating
- Confusion
- Slow or slurred speech

Emotional
- Irritability
- Mood swings
- Sudden crying or anger

Mental symptoms of hypoglycemia can be more serious than physical symptoms because they can prevent the person with diabetes from recognizing that there is a problem and doing something about it.

While most people with diabetes experience the classic symptoms of hypoglycemia, you can't rely on symptoms to warn of low blood sugar. You must test your blood sugar regularly.

If you think you may be low, test your blood sugar and then treat the low. On a number of occasions, my daughter has said she felt low, only to test and find that her blood sugar was in the normal or high range. You may feel sweaty and shaky before a business meeting or speech, not because you're low but because you're experiencing the classic physical responses to adrenaline. Bottom line: You can't really be sure of your blood sugar level unless you test it.

How Hypoglycemia Works

Your body is designed to resist hypoglycemia. When your blood sugar dips, the body releases hormones that cause the liver to dump sugar into the bloodstream. These hormones include glucagon, cortisol, growth hormone, and adrenaline. The physical symptoms of hypoglycemia—the empty, clammy, shaky feeling—are similar to the feeling of an adrenaline rush, the "fight or flight" response that follows the release of adrenaline.

The mental symptoms of hypoglycemia are caused by diminished circulation of sugar to the brain. When blood sugar falls too low, the brain does not function properly. Fortunately, when the blood sugar level returns to normal, brain function is restored, typically within minutes.

In episodes of severe hypoglycemia, the brain is starved for glucose and the hormone response is insufficient. The body responds by going into a seizure, which literally squeezes out the glycogen—sugar—stored in the muscles. While the thought of having a seizure may be frightening, the seizure itself is a lifesaving protective response. Many diabetics who have had seizures report that they feel fine moments after regaining consciousness.

One of the major problems with severe hypoglycemia is that you may lose the ability to act on your own behalf. During episodes of mild or moderate hypoglycemia, you have the ability to test and consume sugar on your own. During episodes of severe hypoglycemia, someone else must assist you to avoid a seizure or coma.

In very rare cases, episodes of hypoglycemia can be fatal, although the problems typically arise from accidents and injuries that occur during the low. For example, someone might go low and cause a traffic accident, experience a fall, or aspirate fluid during a seizure.

Preventing Hypoglycemia

Hypoglycemia is caused by too little food, too much insulin, too much exercise, or a combination of these factors. Keep these key concepts in mind to avoid lows.

Don't try to keep your blood sugar so low that you experience frequent episodes of hypoglycemia. If you strive for excellent control, you are more vulnerable to blood sugar lows because you have a smaller margin of error than you would if you allowed your blood sugar to run a bit higher. The tighter you control your blood sugar, the more important it is for you to be aware of the warning signs of hypoglycemia.

Try to keep an eye out for patterns in your lows. If you experience lows at the same time of day, for example, you will want to relax your control at that time of day. If you're facing a sporting event, a long plane flight, a long drive, or another situation where experiencing a low may be especially difficult or dangerous, you may want to allow your blood sugar to go a little higher than normal until you're back in your regular routine.

Learn to predict how your body handles insulin. Taking too much insulin—especially too much fast-acting insulin—is one of the major causes of hypoglycemia.

There may also be factors that affect the absorption of insulin:

- Injecting insulin or placing an infusion in a place with scar tissue may cause erratic absorption of the medication.

- Exercise in the muscle where you injected insulin can cause more rapid absorption and hypoglycemia.

- Switching to a new bottle of insulin can provide extra kick, which can possibly cause low blood sugar.

Count carbohydrates carefully, and never miss a meal. Incorrectly estimating the amount of carbohydrates in your meal, skipping meals, or eating later than normal can also cause low blood sugar.

Be aware of the impact of exercise on your blood sugar. Exercising more than usual can cause low blood sugar. While you need carbohydrates during exercise to avoid low blood sugar, you can experience a decline in blood sugar for as much as 24 hours after exercise. You need to have a convenient source of sugar during the time you are exercising, and you probably want to wake up at 2 or 3 A.M. to test your sugar during the night. During exercise, your body uses the sugar stored as glycogen in the muscles; in the overnight hours, the muscles draw sugar from the bloodstream to restore the glycogen, causing the possible low blood sugar. (For more information about managing blood sugar during exercise, see Chapter 12.)

Avoid alcohol. Drinking alcohol—even just two or three ounces—can cause hypoglycemia because the alcohol interferes with the release of glucose from the liver. If you plan to consume alcohol, always eat first so you will have some carbohydrate in your system. Test your blood sugar before and after consuming alcohol, and do not overindulge. Some of the symptoms of hypoglycemia can mimic those of intoxication, making it difficult for those around you to recognize that your blood sugar may be dangerously low. (For more information on alcohol, see Chapter 10.)

Watch for signs of hypoglycemia if you are taking oral diabetes medications. While hypoglycemia is most common among people taking insulin, it does occur in people with type 2 diabetes who take oral medications as well.

Test your blood sugar often if you're taking beta blockers. Prescription beta blockers, used to treat high blood pressure and heart disease, can interfere with some of the physical warning signs of hypoglycemia. If you take these drugs, test your blood sugar regularly and do not rely on the physical warning signs of hypoglycemia to remind you to test.

Be aware of your menstrual cycle, if you are a woman. Your insulin demands change during different phases of your menstrual cycle. Typically, the need for insulin increases several days before a woman's period begins, then declines suddenly when bleeding begins, leaving a woman prone to hypoglycemia if she continues taking the higher dose of insulin medication. The erratic blood sugar levels reflect fluctuations in the amount of the hormone progesterone in the body; progesterone makes insulin less effective. Women should try to learn the patterns of their cycles so that they can anticipate the changes in insulin demand.

Hypoglycemic Unawareness

One of the most important ways of avoiding dangerous bouts of hypoglycemia is to be aware of how you are feeling at all times and test your blood sugar whenever you think you may be going low. Unfortunately, some people with diabetes develop hypoglycemic unawareness, meaning they lose the ability to recognize when their blood sugar is dipping too low. Without warning, people with hypoglycemic unawareness become so low that they are unable to care for themselves, either because they can't think clearly or because they lose consciousness.

Gladys, who had type 1 diabetes for nearly 50 years, developed hypoglycemic unawareness when she was in her late fifties. "I could be walking down the hallway and suddenly fall over without warning," Gladys said. "It was unexpected. That's what made it so frightening."

Gladys's condition eventually reached the point where her diabetes was life-threatening, and she received a pancreas/kidney transplant. While she is on immunosuppressive drugs—and will be for the rest of her life—she is technically no longer diabetic.

Hypoglycemic unawareness occurs most often in people like Gladys who have had diabetes for 15 or 20 years or longer. It usually starts with a decline in symptoms as the body becomes less able to recognize signs of low blood sugar. The condition is caused by nerve damage to the sensors that release the hormone adrenaline, which, as mentioned earlier, raises blood sugar and triggers the classic hypoglycemic symptoms. Instead of experiencing the sweating and trembling and other physical signs of hypoglycemia, your blood sugar continues to go down until your brain is in dire need of sugar and you experience confusion and signs of mental impairment. This is particularly dangerous because at this point it becomes much more difficult for you to treat the problem on your own.

Wild fluctuations in blood sugar make the problems worse. Likewise, maintaining excellent control through frequent testing helps to calm the system and improve the ability to detect lows.

Blood glucose awareness training can help people recognize when their blood sugar is dropping. This is a system for teaching people to identify and treat low blood sugars at the earliest stages. Ask your doctor about blood glucose awareness training if you have problems identifying when you are at risk of hypoglycemia.

Hypoglycemia and Children

It can be especially difficult for some children to identify when they are low. Sometimes at lunch my daughter's blood sugar would be in the 50s or 60s and I would ask if she felt low. When she stopped to think about it, she admitted that she did feel kind of low, but she wanted to finish what she was doing. It took quite a while to teach her to tune into her body and to take steps to deal with her diabetes whenever she felt that she might be high or low.

To help her become more aware of how her body was feeling, we also made up a game we call High-Low-Jackpot. Before testing I ask her if she is high (above 180), low (below 80), or jackpot (in between). This game helped her to learn to focus on what her body was telling

Contra Costa County Library
Ygnacio Valley
9/24/2019 6:40:19 PM

- Patron Receipt -
- Charges -

ID: 21901024243077

Item: 31901052130293
Title: The complete guide to living well with dia
Call Number: 616.462 CONKLING
Due Date: 10/15/2019

All Contra Costa County Libraries will be
closed on Monday, October 14th and
Monday, November 11th. Items may be
renewed at ccclib.org or by calling
1-800-984-4636, menu option 1. Book drops
will be open. El Sobrante Library remains
closed for repairs.

her about her blood sugar, and the immediate feedback of her actual number helped her identify which feelings were associated with the highs and lows.

Treating Hypoglycemia

To treat hypoglycemia, eat. Sounds simple enough, but it can be tricky to consume the right amount of carbohydrates, so you don't end up too high or too low after treatment.

You never know when hypoglycemia will strike, so you should *always* have a source of sugar with you. Keep juice boxes, glucose tablets, or another simple carbohydrate in the car, by the bed, in your purse, in your desk at work, or anywhere you may need them.

Don't ignore the first warning signs that you may be low. Test and treat a low, even if you're planning to eat in a half hour or so. A small problem can become a big one if you don't pay attention to the symptoms.

On the other hand, don't overreact to the low and eat your way into high blood sugar that will need to be treated with insulin. Keep in mind that it usually takes about 15 minutes for the food or drink you consume to have an impact on your blood sugar. To avoid overtreating a low, consume about 15 grams of carbohydrate and wait 15 minutes to retest. If your blood sugar is still below 60, consume another 15 grams of carbohydrate and then test again.

Examples of fast-acting 15-gram carbohydrate snacks include:

4 to 6 ounces of juice or regular soda
2 or 3 glucose tablets (5 grams each)
6 saltine crackers
3 graham crackers

15 Skittles candies
5 Life Savers candies
$\frac{1}{3}$ cup raisins

If you opt for candies or fruit, be sure to chew your food thoroughly to break it down and make it easier to digest. Don't eat ice cream, chocolates, or other foods that contain fat, which can slow the absorption of the carbohydrates.

Managing Severe Hypoglycemia with Glucagon

If you experience severe hypoglycemia, you can't care for yourself. That's why it's always important that you let your family members and coworkers know about your diabetes and how to handle an episode of low blood sugar. The essential rules are:

- No one should ever put food or drink in your mouth unless you are sitting up and able to swallow.

- If you cannot swallow, the person with you should dial 9-1-1 and then administer Glucagon, if it is available.

Glucagon should only be used if the person with diabetes is unresponsive or unconscious. Glucagon is a naturally occurring hormone that will increase blood sugar in case of emergency. Glucagon must be injected into the muscle (typically the thigh or shoulder muscle). It comes in a kit with instructions, but ideally your family, friends, and coworkers should know where you keep it and be able to use it if you need it. It isn't difficult to do, but it requires practice, especially for people unfamiliar with needles.

Most people feel nauseated or vomit after receiving Glucagon, so they should be turned on their side to avoid swallowing or inhaling vomit. They should not be left alone. Also, you or someone with you should test your blood sugar every 30 to 60 minutes after you receive Glucagon to make sure that your low blood sugar does not return.

Glucagon should be kept at home, at school, at work, and anywhere else you keep diabetic supplies. It comes as a kit—a small plastic case with a vial of powdered hormone, a vial of fluid, and a sterile syringe. The powder must be mixed with the liquid and drawn into the syringe. Keep in mind that the shelf life of a Glucagon kit is about one year, so you should check the expiration dates and replace your kits on a regular basis.

As soon as you regain consciousness, you should eat something with carbohydrates that is easy to digest, such as sugared soda and crackers. The food is necessary to replenish the glucose in the liver. After 15 minutes, test your blood sugar and eat a more significant meal, such as a sandwich and milk.

Even small children who may not be able to administer Glucagon should be taught how to dial 9-1-1 in an emergency. Children as young as three and four years old routinely save their parents' lives by calling for help when a diabetic parent passes out or is unable to care for himself.

Overnight Hypoglycemia

More than half of all cases of severe hypoglycemia occur in the night because when you're asleep, you're not aware that you're going low. To avoid overnight hypoglycemia, test your blood sugar before going to bed and eat a snack if your blood sugar is less than 120.

Many people with diabetes wake up between 2 and 3 A.M. to test their blood sugar, a time frame in which many people experience lows. Some doctors recommend abandoning this overnight check, while others think it's a good habit. (I check my daughter every night at 2 A.M.—and even more often if she has had a particularly active day.) Even if you don't do an overnight test every night, it's a good idea to spot-check every couple of weeks so that you can assess how your blood sugar levels are doing in the overnight hours.

Hypoglycemia is a common challenge for people with diabetes, but by paying careful attention to your symptoms, you can deal with most episodes before the problem becomes dangerous. Any time you are suspicious of your blood sugar level, take two minutes out of your day to test. Always have a source of sugar with you, so that you can respond to a blood sugar low promptly.

While hypoglycemia can occur in people with either type 1 or type 2 diabetes, it is most common among people taking insulin. The following chapter will discuss the various types of insulin and how to use them safely.

CHAPTER 7
INSULIN

Charles had managed his type 2 diabetes for years by watching his diet and taking oral medications. When his blood sugar levels began running high, he assumed he could control the problem by tightening his diet even more. When that didn't work and his doctor told him he needed to take insulin, he was distraught: He felt as if he had failed to manage his diabetes on his own. It took a long time for his doctor to convince Charles that he was doing a laudable job of disease management and the best thing he could do for his health was to begin taking insulin to maintain his good control.

"I thought I could handle my diabetes," Charles said. "When I had to take insulin, I felt like I had failed. At that point, the disease won."

Other people, such as Ruth, have no problem accepting that they need to take insulin. She had to adjust to giving herself injections, but she did not have a psychological barrier to overcome when she began to use insulin. "Once I got used to the idea of having diabetes, I always assumed I would need insulin," Ruth said. "My mother needed insulin, so I figured sooner or later I would, too."

Taking insulin can be a very emotional issue for some people. But before you bemoan the need to take the drug, it may help you to realize that before insulin was available, most people with type 1 diabetes died within a year of diagnosis. The first patient to receive insulin—a 14-year-old boy in Toronto—lived 13 more years by taking what could only be described by people at the time as a miracle drug.

How Insulin Works

No one can live without insulin. If your body can't make enough of the hormone, you need to take extra. Insulin allows the body to use sugar in the blood as fuel for the cells. Sugar in the blood comes directly from the carbohydrates you consume as food and indirectly from the liver.

Insulin helps control blood sugar in several ways:

- Insulin increases the removal of glucose from the blood.

- Insulin allows the cells to use the sugar floating around in the blood as fuel.

- Insulin signals the liver to stop producing extra sugar.

- Insulin helps build muscle by delivering amino acids to the muscles. Without enough insulin, the amino acids are used by the liver for glucose formation.

- Insulin encourages the body to store extra calories as fat and glycogen. Too little insulin causes uncontrolled weight loss—and ketoacidosis (explained in Chapter 15).

• Insulin is essential in the hormonal changes of menstruation.

Because insulin plays such a vital role in so many essential bodily processes, you might assume that people would willingly take it if their bodies needed it. Taking insulin probably wouldn't be such a big deal, except that it is given by injection or insulin pump infusion (which also involves needles). Insulin pumps are discussed in the following chapter, but even people who use pumps must sometimes receive insulin by injection.

Daily injections of insulin can be quite intimidating for many people. Keep in mind that insulin needles are very sharp, fine, and coated with silicone so they can slip in and out almost painlessly. That said, there is still a psychological hurdle to overcome, and different people handle the stress of learning how to administer injections differently. Ultimately, almost everyone learns to manage injections without too much stress. Nurse educators and your endocrinologist should be able to help you learn to give injections with minimal anxiety.

In addition to needle phobia, many people taking insulin fear the possibility of hypoglycemia (discussed in the previous chapter). Some people also feel overwhelmed by the burden of taking insulin every day for the rest of their lives. Diabetes requires attention 24/7, forever—or until there's a cure.

Some people with type 2 diabetes feel that their diabetes is "worse" than someone else's if they need to take insulin and the other person does not. Rather than using insulin as a dividing line—better on one side, worse on the other—focus on the ultimate goal: good overall health without complications caused by your diabetes. If taking insulin can help you reach that goal, then you're better off using it than you would be by avoiding it. Your goal is good control, and insulin is just a tool used to achieve that goal.

Often people with type 2 diabetes want to try to exercise and lose weight while taking oral diabetes medication to see if they can bring their blood sugar down to an acceptable level without taking insulin. If you're able to change your lifestyle and reach your blood sugar goals with your doctor's approval, then terrific. In some circumstances doctors give their patients a month or so to try to see if they can lower their blood sugar on their own, but if your blood sugar is still too high after doing your best to make lifestyle adjustments, consider taking insulin. Again, the goal is good blood sugar control, and you should use all the resources available to you to reach that goal.

Insulin and Type 1 Diabetes

Everyone with type 1 diabetes needs to take insulin. Most people start taking insulin as soon as they are diagnosed with the condition.

As mentioned earlier, many people with type 1 diabetes go through a phase known as the "honeymoon" when the pancreas seems to recover somewhat and the person has good control with minimal insulin use. This period can last from several months to a year or so, but alas, it eventually passes. During the honeymoon, the beta cells of the pancreas rally for a time, although the immune system is continuing to destroy the remaining beta cells. In time, the immune system wins the battle and the honeymoon is over.

If you're in a honeymoon period, enjoy it. I remember when my daughter started on insulin and she had stable numbers with good control, I felt delighted with her progress. I knew we were in the honeymoon period, but emotionally I needed the encouragement that first period provided. During that window, I was able to learn about diabetes and become familiar with using insulin while the disease was a bit easier to control. As I felt more competent, the disease became trickier, but I felt a bit more prepared to face the challenges.

When the honeymoon period is over, you are effectively required to think like a pancreas by learning how to juggle and balance insulin, carbohydrates, and exercise to keep blood sugars in your target range. Fine-tuning these variables isn't easy, but it is the essence of diabetic control. Over time, you will learn how your body responds to various conditions, and, believe it or not, many of the decisions you will need to make will become second nature.

Insulin and Type 2 Diabetes

Calling type 2 diabetes "non-insulin-dependent diabetes" is a misnomer. Many people with type 2 diabetes need insulin to maintain good blood sugar control. The problem is not with the diagnosis but with the name.

Your doctor will know if you need insulin to control your type 2 diabetes. As a general rule, you need supplemental insulin if your pancreas isn't strong enough to keep up with your body's demands for insulin. The warning signs are the same as they are for type 1 diabetes—high blood sugar, weight loss, thirst, and frequent urination. Some people with type 2 diabetes recognize these symptoms after they have tried to control the disease with diet, exercise, and oral medications. Some people attempt to exercise more or eat less to avoid insulin, but it doesn't make sense to strive for an unrealistic lifestyle that can't be sustained for the long haul.

For type 2 diabetics, insulin is meant to supplement the body's existing insulin, so it is usually easier to achieve good control than it is for type 1 diabetics. Most people need only one or two injections daily. Ironically, many type 2 diabetics end up taking more units of insulin than type 1 diabetics—sometimes 50 to 100 units a day for large people. In other words, a person with type 2 diabetes who is very insulin resistant may need more units of insulin each day than a person with type 1 diabetes who is not insulin resistant.

In addition, some people need insulin only temporarily, such as during pregnancy or periods of high stress. Since women who develop gestational diabetes cannot take oral diabetes medications, they must use insulin to lower their blood sugar. After the baby is born, most women with gestational diabetes no longer need insulin, although they are at increased risk of developing type 2 diabetes later. (For more information on gestational diabetes, see Chapter 13.)

People with type 2 diabetes may need to take insulin when they recover from surgery or go through a particularly stressful period. When the person has recovered, insulin may no longer be necessary.

Reactions to Insulin

While insulin is a lifesaving miracle drug to those who need it, it can have unpleasant side effects for some people in some circumstances.

Weight gain: When you are taking the right amount of insulin and your blood sugar is under control, your body uses all of the calories you consume, rather than spilling some of them into your urine. If you consume extra calories, the surplus is stored as fat, just as it is in people without diabetes. To avoid unneeded calories, adjust your insulin dose to avoid hypoglycemia, which is treated with extra calories. (For more on hypoglycemia, see Chapter 6.)

Insulin allergy: Although rare, insulin can cause an allergic reaction in diabetics. Some people experience a local insulin allergy (redness and possible itching around the injection site) or a systemic allergy (hives, rashes away from the injection site, swelling, and wheezing). Local reactions are rarely severe. Systemic reactions can be more dangerous, so you will need to work with your endocrinologist and allergist to use insulin safely.

Insulin edema: Some diabetics who had very poor insulin control before taking insulin develop swelling or edema when they begin using insulin. The situation usually resolves within a few weeks. If necessary, your doctor may prescribe a diuretic and a low-sodium diet during this transition period.

Types of Insulin

The first insulin was made from cow and pig pancreases, but in the 1980s drug companies developed human insulin using DNA technology. It is made by bacteria that have been altered to make insulin exactly like human insulin, so it causes fewer allergic reactions. The two manufacturers of human insulin are Humulin (Eli Lilly) and Novolin (Novo Nordisk).

Measuring Insulin

Insulin is measured in standardized units. One unit of insulin lowers the blood sugar by a fixed amount, although that amount varies from person to person. When you begin to take insulin, your doctor will work with you to determine how much one unit of insulin lowers your blood sugar. This number will help you determine how much insulin you need to take to cover the food you are eating.

For example, if one unit of insulin lowers your blood sugar by the same amount that 15 grams of carbohydrates would raise your blood sugar, then you would need three units of insulin to cover 45 grams of carbohydrates. Using this information, you will count the number of carbohydrates you eat, and cover that by taking the number of units of insulin necessary to lower your blood sugar by the same amount. (For more information on counting carbohydrates, see Chapter 10.)

In the United States, insulin is concentrated as 100 units per milliliter or U-100. In other countries, concentrations of U-40 or 40 units per milliliter are common. If you plan to travel overseas, take extra U-100 insulin with you to avoid confusion.

Insulin syringes come in several sizes, depending on the amount of insulin you take. If you take large doses, such as 80 units at a time, you need a syringe large enough to hold 100 units of U-100 insulin. For people who take smaller doses, syringes are calibrated to hold 30 or 50 units. The smaller the amount, the greater the accuracy in measuring. Your doctor will prescribe the correct size needles for your insulin needs.

Comparing Types of Insulin

Insulin doesn't start working the minute it is injected. It takes time for it to make its way into the cells and to reach maximum effectiveness. Different types of insulin are formulated to have different periods of effectiveness. When comparing insulin products, the time period of action is measured in three ways:

- Onset, or how quickly the insulin begins to work

- Peak, or the point at which insulin is most potent

- Duration, or how long the insulin lowers blood sugar

While the drug manufacturers formulate their products to have certain characteristics, your body may respond differently to the products. For example, one person may find that a product has a duration of four hours, while in another person it remains effective for six hours. Your doctor will be able to work with you to determine how your body handles insulin. This is important to understand so that you do not inadvertently take a dose of insulin and then take a second dose before the first has worn off. Taking insulin too close together can create a situation known as "stacking," which can cause hypoglycemia.

There are a number of types of insulin:

Rapid-Acting (Humalog or Lispro)
- Onset: About 10 minutes
- Peak: About 1 hour
- Duration: 2 to 4 hours

Short-Acting (Regular)
- Onset: 30 to 45 minutes
- Peak: About 2 hours
- Duration: 4 to 6 hours

Intermediate-Acting (NPH—Neutral Protamine Hagedorn—or Lente)
- Onset: 1 hour
- Peak: 6 to 8 hours
- Duration: 12 to 18 hours

These intermediate-acting insulins are absorbed more slowly because of the addition of proteins (NPH) or changes in the size of the insulin crystals (Lente).

Long-Acting (Ultralente)
- Onset: Slow
- Peak: 8 to 12 hours
- Duration: Up to 36 hours

Regular insulin is clear. Intermediate- and long-acting insulins are cloudy. The insulin is actually in the particles, so the bottle must be gently mixed before the insulin is used.

Many people use more than one type of insulin during the course of the day. Be sure to look at the product labels carefully to avoid confusion.

Some forms of insulin are marketed as a combination of NPH and regular, such as 70/30 or 70 percent NPH and 30 percent regular. You can also mix your own by drawing insulin from two different bottles before administering the injection. (This process is discussed below.)

Treating Your Insulin Right

Insulin is a fragile protein that needs special handling to maintain its potency:

- Handle with care. Don't vigorously shake insulin. Instead, roll the vial back and forth with the palms of your hands to mix it prior to use. Too much shaking can damage the proteins.

- Avoid extreme heat or cold. Insulin can be left out at room temperature, but most doctors and pharmacists recommend storing it in a refrigerator, not a freezer. (In our household we store the insulin in the butter drawer of the refrigerator.) It should not get hotter than 86 degrees or colder than 40 degrees. Avoid closed cars in summer heat or winter cold. If you're heading for the beach or ski slopes, slip the vial of insulin into an insulated pouch to maintain the appropriate temperature.

- When flying, keep your insulin and other diabetes supplies with you in a carry-on. The cargo area can have extremes in temperature, and you can't be confident that your bags will join you at your destination.

Sometimes insulin goes bad, either because it isn't handled properly or for other unknown reasons. You may suspect bad insulin if it is ineffective—your blood sugar remains high after you administer insulin and there is no apparent reason why. Some people notice that their insulin seems to have less kick by the time they reach the bottom of the bottle. If you experience this, discard the remaining insulin and open a new vial.

Examine your insulin before using it. If clear insulin becomes cloudy or cloudy insulin becomes clumpy, then discard it and switch to a new bottle. Always keep an unopened vial of insulin in the refrigerator so that it is available if one bottle goes bad, or if you accidentally break it at midnight of a holiday weekend when all the pharmacies are closed.

Using Insulin

Okay, this is the part many people fear—the needles. But after you inject insulin a couple of times, it will become second nature to you. That is not a line written casually: I was fairly needle-phobic until the day my daughter developed diabetes. I gave her the first injection of insulin, not because I wanted to, but because I felt I had no choice. I no longer had the luxury of feeling squeamish about needles.

If you have diabetes and need insulin, you may be surprised that you can do more than you ever imagined possible to take care of yourself. You are blessed to have insulin and sterile needles and other medical supplies available to you. With your doctor's help, you can discover the reserves of courage within yourself and overcome any anxiety you may have about injecting insulin.

Once you overcome any psychological obstacles about needles and syringes, you will probably find that injecting insulin isn't as daunting a task as it seems.

- Wash your hands with soap and water.

- Lay out all of your supplies: vial of insulin, alcohol wipes, a clean syringe.

- Wipe the rubber stopper on the top of the insulin vial with an alcohol wipe.

- Wipe the surface of your skin where you plan to do the injection with an alcohol wipe.

- If you are using cloudy insulin—NPH, Lente, or long-acting insulin—roll the bottle back and forth in the palms of your hands to mix the contents thoroughly. Don't shake.

- Draw back the plunger of the syringe to displace the same amount of air as insulin that you need. Stick the needle through the rubber stopper on the insulin bottle and inject the air into the vial. (This will make it easier to withdraw the insulin because it prevents a vacuum from forming inside the insulin bottle.)

- Turn the vial upside down so that the tip of the needle is covered with insulin.

- Pull back the plunger, drawing insulin into the syringe. Take a little bit more than you need, then tap the syringe to loosen any air bubbles and force them to the top. Push the extra insulin and air bubble out of the top of the syringe and back into the bottle. When the plunger is at the desired mark, withdraw the syringe. (Don't panic about tiny air bubbles. Air bubbles in the veins are dangerous, but you will be injecting into the fatty layer. You want to minimize air because air bubbles mean you aren't getting all the insulin you need.)

- Pinch the skin and quickly insert the needle. Push down the plunger, release the pinch, and withdraw the needle.

- Dispose of the used syringe in a sharps container. Never reuse or share syringes because of the risk of infection.

If your doctor recommends that you mix two different forms of insulin—such as a short-acting insulin and a long-acting insulin—you will need to add a couple of steps in order to combine the insulin in a single syringe. You don't want the additives in the longer-acting insulin to contaminate the regular insulin. To prevent contamination, displace the air from the cloudy bottle, then remove the syringe without withdrawing any insulin. Next, displace the air from the clear bottle and withdraw the clear insulin. Insert the needle into the cloudy bottle and withdraw the additional insulin. (At this point, you can't put any insulin back into the bottle, so you need to withdraw the insulin carefully.) Then do the injection.

This sounds complicated, but it will become second nature. At first I thought I'd just give two separate shots, but I didn't want to put my daughter through the extra injections. I reminded myself every time I did an injection, "Cloudy, clear—clear, cloudy." By customizing the fast- and slower-acting insulin mixture, you will be able to have better blood sugar control, so it will be worth the effort to figure out how to mix insulin, if your doctor recommends it.

Insulin Pens

An insulin pen holds insulin in a cartridge similar to the cartridge in a fountain pen. Instead of a nib, the pen has a disposable needle at the tip. Some pens are completely disposable; others have refillable cartridges.

Insulin pens are simple and easy to use. They have a dial to determine the number of units to be administered. Using insulin pens, most people—including children—can administer insulin accurately in half-unit increments.

Not only are they easy to use, but insulin pens can be slipped into a pocket or purse and used with discretion. Michelle carried her insulin pen with her to the high school homecoming dance. When she was at dinner with friends, she ordered her meal and then dialed the amount and jabbed the pen into her thigh right through her dress. Most of the people at the table had no idea she was giving herself an insulin injection.

"It's not really such a big deal," Michelle said. "A lot of my friends didn't even know I had diabetes."

Where to Inject Insulin

Insulin is injected into the fatty tissue in the arms, legs, buttocks, and stomach (at least 2 inches away from the belly button). You will almost certainly discover that different areas lead to different rates of insulin absorption. Typically, insulin is absorbed fastest in the abdomen, slowest in the buttocks, and in between in the arms and legs. With my daughter, we found about an hour difference in the absorption rate between the abdomen and buttocks, so we often tried to inject into the abdomen when she was high and needed the insulin fast and into the buttocks when she was running a bit low and could wait a bit for the insulin to kick in.

You need to rotate injection sites so that you don't overuse one particular area. My daughter prefers her lower abdomen and would have all her insulin there if we let her. Using the same site too often can cause fatty deposits to form under the skin, which can cause problems with absorption.

Consider your planned activity when you decide where to inject insulin. Avoid injecting insulin into your legs if you're about to exercise, since the use of the muscle can cause the insulin to be absorbed too quickly. In other words, don't give yourself a shot in the thigh and then head out for a 2-mile run or you may experience a sudden rush of insulin and an episode of hypoglycemia.

Different Insulin Plans

Different types of insulin can be used in any number of combinations to address certain challenges. Some of the common approaches include the following:

- Bedtime insulin, daytime medication: People with type 2 diabetes who have high blood sugar despite the use of oral medication sometimes find it helpful to take a bedtime dose of insulin to lower blood sugar overnight. They then use oral medication during the day.

- Two injections a day: People with type 1 diabetes may take two shots a day, combining regular and intermediate-acting insulin in both injections. Breakfast is covered by the regular insulin in the morning injection, and lunch is covered by the intermediate-acting insulin in the morning injection. Dinner is covered by the regular insulin in the night-time injection, and the overnight hours are covered by the intermediate-acting insulin.

- Intensive insulin regimen: People with type 1 diabetes who strive for tight control sometimes use one dose of long-acting insulin once a day, along with injections of regular insulin to cover every meal.

There are any number of combinations of insulin that can be used to customize an approach that works for you. You'll need to carefully monitor and record your blood sugar levels throughout the day to determine when your blood sugar levels tend to rise and fall. Using this information, you and your doctor can design an insulin strategy that works for your lifestyle, eating pattern, and tolerance for medication. Again, there is not one right or wrong way to design your program. Your goal should simply be excellent blood sugar control.

Stay Flexible

One of the most exasperating things about dealing with diabetes is that your work is never done. Once you figure out the perfect insulin regimen, something in your life or your body changes and you need to make adjustments in your dosing. Don't fight it; accept it. You just need to know enough about your diabetes to be able to stay flexible and adapt to the changes.

While you want all of your blood sugar readings to be on target, don't fret if one number is wildly out of line. On the other hand, if you test regularly and detect a pattern in your blood sugar, then you need to make an adjustment in your routine. For example, if you notice that you're low before lunch four times in a single week, you're going to need to scale back on the insulin dose at breakfast.

My daughter's endocrinologist has her use two different colored highlighters and go through her records highlighting highs in one color and lows in another. Patterns of unwanted highs and lows visually pop off the page, making it very clear where the problems lie and when adjustments in insulin levels need to be made.

Many doctors create a sliding scale for their patients so that they can adjust their insulin dose with every injection. The scale takes into account your current blood sugar level and recommends a dose based on that number. The higher your blood sugar level, the greater the amount of insulin you would receive. Again, you will need to test often and keep good records to identify trends and make the necessary adjustments.

Don't make dramatic changes in your insulin routine at any one time. As a general rule, don't change your dose by more than 10 to 20 percent at a time, and don't change it more than every three or four days. You need to give yourself enough time to recognize patterns so that you can adjust to them.

If you're ever unsure of how to make an adjustment, talk to your doctor. You and your doctor are a team, and together you can work toward the goal of excellent blood sugar control.

While many people with diabetes learn to work with injections and stick with that approach for insulin delivery, others find that using an insulin pump provides more flexibility in their daily routines. Insulin pumps are discussed in detail in the following chapter.

CHAPTER 8
INSULIN PUMPS

Less than a year after my daughter was diagnosed with type 1 diabetes, her endocrinologist sponsored a clinic on insulin pumps. Three or four pump manufacturers presented their products and explained the benefits of pump technology. While I was hesitant to send my daughter to second grade with an expensive piece of medical machinery attached to her waistband, I was convinced that the pump would give her more flexibility to eat and play like the other kids in her class. One year later, I can't imagine going back to daily injections—and neither can she.

Some people prefer insulin pumps because they make it much easier to eat what you want when you want. There's no need to "feed the insulin" and eat mandatory meals at fixed times to avoid hypoglycemia. Most pumps can be worn for about three days before you need to replace the infusion set, so there are significantly fewer needles to fuss with. For routine outings less than a couple of hours from home, there's no need to bring a diabetes kit equipped with syringes and insulin and alcohol wipes.

On the other hand, some people with diabetes can't tolerate insulin pumps. They can't stand to be attached to a device, and they don't want the external reminder of their diabetes worn on their bodies all the time. Some refuse to try the pump because they worry that the technology will fail or malfunction, causing serious medical harm.

Connie tried switching to an insulin pump on two separate occasions. "I could never get the hang of it," said the 32-year-old type 1 diabetic. "I find injections much easier to deal with." She has excellent control and has decided to stick with the system that is working for her.

What Is an Insulin Pump?

An insulin pump is an external device about the size of a pager that can be clipped to a waistband or slipped into a pocket. It contains a reservoir filled with insulin that is administered in a slow, steady drip. A long thin plastic tube runs from the pump to an infusion set, which looks like a small bandage attached to the skin. A short plastic cannula remains under the skin, allowing the insulin to trickle into the layer of fat under the skin. The cannula remains under the skin for two or three days, but the tubing can be detached for showering and swimming.

The technology behind the insulin pump is called "open loop," meaning that the pump can't think for itself. You need to test your blood sugar and tell it how many carbohydrates you plan to consume, and the pump will recommend a dose of insulin. You then have to accept the dose and tell the pump to give you the insulin. "Closed loop" technology involves pumps that will test your blood sugar and administer the insulin on their own. These devices are available only in research trials at this time.

One hybrid product available from several pump

manufacturers combines a traditional open loop system
with a continuous glucose monitor. These devices constantly update your blood sugar level, but you still need to
confirm the reading with a finger-stick before giving insulin. This is the system we chose for my daughter. The
continuous glucose monitor can be programmed to alarm
when her blood sugar is high or low, so I am more comfortable trusting that we will catch any episodes of hypoglycemia or hyperglycemia before they become problems.
(Continuous glucose monitors are discussed in Chapter 5.)

How Insulin Pumps Work

Insulin pumps are loaded with short-acting insulin, which
is delivered at two rates:

- Basal rate: A slow continuous drip that provides
  the background level of insulin.

- The bolus: A faster surge of insulin to cover the
  food you eat, or to correct blood sugar if levels
  are too high.

Your doctor will help you program your pump and set
the initial rates, although it will need to be fine-tuned
many times. The basal or background rate typically ac-
counts for about 40 percent of the total amount of insulin taken over a 24-hour period. If the basal rate is
accurate, your blood sugar level should remain flat during the times you are not eating. If the rate drifts up, you
need a higher basal rate; if it drifts down, you need a
lower basal rate.

The bolus dose is based on how much your blood sugar

drops after taking a unit of insulin. Using this information, the pump will recommend how much insulin you need to reach your target blood sugar level. Most pumps ask for a current blood sugar reading and the amount of carbohydrates you plan to consume in grams; then the pump indicates how much insulin you need. You can decide to take the bolus all at once, or you can extend the bolus over a period of time. (This can be helpful if you are eating a high-fat meal that will be absorbed over a number of hours.)

Why Should You Consider a Pump?

Pump technology offers several advantages over traditional injections:

- Flexibility: People with diabetes who take injections need to eat approximately the same number of carbohydrates at the same time each day. With a pump, you can eat lunch at 11 A.M. or 2 P.M., or you can skip it altogether and your blood sugar level should remain balanced.

- Insulin limits: Pumps are programmed with maximum bolus and basal rates so that you cannot accidentally deliver too much insulin.

- Alarms: Insulin pumps have alarms that sound if insulin isn't passing through the tube or if the reservoir holding the insulin runs low.

- Improved blood sugar control: Evidence indicates that most people using external insulin pumps are able to control their blood sugar better than those taking insulin by injection. Diabetics must still monitor their blood sugar and learn to make adjustments in the pump, but if they're attentive to using the technology, most people can obtain good control. The pump can also reduce the chances of uncomfortable blood sugar swings because the insulin is released in a pattern that more closely resembles that of a healthy pancreas.

On the other hand, pump therapy is not without its problems:

• Skin infections: Because the cannula remains under the skin for several days, there is a greater risk of skin infection than with injections. Infections, which look something in between a pimple and a boil, tend to affect some people more than others; if you're susceptible to local skin infection, you should change your infusion sites more frequently.

• Increased risk of diabetic ketoacidosis: Pump malfunctions can put people at risk of developing diabetic ketoacidosis (described in detail in Chapter 15). If you monitor your blood sugar regularly and respond to every pump alarm, you are not likely to develop this complication, but you should be aware that it is more common in people using pump therapy. This problem most often arises when the pump reservoir is empty and the person fails to heed the low reservoir alarm.

Other problems include the cannula falling out or a kink in the tubing, but each of the problems should be detected early if you do regular blood sugar monitoring.

• Expense: Insulin pumps and supplies are quite expensive, even when the bulk of the expense is covered by insurance. Diabetes is an expensive disease, and if finances are a significant issue, you should ask your insurance company to compare the annual out-of-pocket costs of injections and pump therapy for you to help you make a decision. (In the long run, the major costs of diabetes involve complications and hospitalizations, which can be avoided with good blood sugar control, making insulin pump therapy a good investment for a person willing to learn to use the device properly.)

• You will be attached to your pump most of the time: Using an insulin pump is a 24/7 commitment. You will take it off to bathe or swim—and some people remove their pump during sex and exercise—but it should remain attached most of the time. (If you remove it for more than an hour or two, you will probably want to compensate with an insulin injection.) Many people don't mind the attachment, but some people don't like the feeling of being attached to a device day and night.

• The device advertises you have diabetes: Wearing an insulin pump invites questions about the device, as well as comments from other people who have diabetes. Some people are very open about their condition, but others prefer to keep their medical issues private. If you wear a pump, you run the risk that other people will see it and recognize it.

If you're interested in using an insulin pump, talk to your doctor. Before trying a pump, you need to be fairly familiar with diabetes, you should be able to count carbohydrates (this is discussed in Chapter 10), and you should be in the habit of checking your blood sugar frequently (at least before every meal and prior to going to bed).

While the devices are fairly easy to use once you become familiar with them, some people can't figure out how to turn on a cell phone, much less program an insulin pump. If you're afraid of technology, then you should look at a number of different pumps to see if one is less intimidating than another and whether you're comfortable with them at all.

Going "Live" with an Insulin Pump

Don't expect to master the pump right away. It can be tricky to get the settings just right, but you don't have to figure it all out by yourself. You should have the support and assistance of your doctor, a pump company trainer, and a nurse educator. Most companies have extensive pump training information on their Web sites as well as 24-hour customer assistance phone numbers.

I was surprised at how long it took to set the basal and bolus rates for the first time; it took several weeks to get the basal adjustments into an acceptable range. That said, the time spent setting the pump was well worth it. Once the rates are set for the first time, it is easier to make minor adjustments.

Before using insulin, many doctors and pump companies will allow you to perform a "saline trial," or a test period in which you become familiar with the pump and how it works, but the pump is filled with salt water rather than insulin. In addition, some companies allow you to try a pump in a saline trial so you can decide how you feel about it before committing to buy one. (Many companies allow potential customers to experience saline trials during diabetes conferences and other diabetes events.)

Once you know how to work all of the settings, you'll go "live" by using your pump with insulin. At this point, you need to determine the correct settings for both the basal and bolus rates. Your doctor will probably recommend a starting basal rate, based on the amount of insulin you were using by injection. (Typically people use less insulin in a pump than they do by injection.) You will need to test your blood sugar often to assess whether the basal rate needs to be adjusted up or down.

Some people stay in the hospital during the initial phase of pump adjustments. Whether you set your pump at home or in the hospital depends on whether you live alone, how stable your blood sugars have been, and what other health problems you may have.

First your doctor and pump team will work on setting the basal rate. Many people have different basal rates at different times of day, just as the body produces different levels of insulin at different times of day. For example, many people need a lower basal rate in the overnight hours than they do during the day. When the rates are set, your blood sugar levels should remain flat in the times that you are not eating or exercising. The secret to setting your basal rate is to test often.

Next, you will focus on the bolus rate, which covers the food you eat and corrects any high blood sugar rates. The goal here is to figure out how much your blood sugar will drop with each unit of insulin. In general, people with high insulin requirements (say, 70 units a day) are not as sensitive to insulin as people with low insulin requirements (less than 30 units a day). Most people have a fairly consistent drop in blood sugar for each unit of insulin they take, although some people are more sensitive at some times of day than others.

When calculating a bolus for food, you will focus on the amount of carbohydrates in the foods you eat. (For more information on carbohydrate counting, see Chapter 10.) The amount of insulin in a bolus is that amount you need to cover the food you eat, plus any correction you need. To calculate the amount, all you have to do is press a few buttons to answer several questions. The pump does the math for you to calculate the exact amount of insulin you need, typically down to the tenth of a unit.

Of course, the body does not respond instantly to the bolus. The bolus releases the insulin, but it usually takes 45 minutes to an hour or longer to see the blood sugar respond to the insulin, just as it would if you gave yourself an injection. To minimize swings in blood sugar, you will need to take your current blood sugar level into account when you decide when to bolus for a meal.

- If your blood sugar level is less than 70, bolus right before eating.

- If your blood sugar level is 70 to 100, bolus 15 minutes before eating.

- If your blood sugar level is 100 to 200, bolus 30 minutes before eating.

- If your blood sugar level is 200 to 300, bolus 45 minutes before eating.

- If your blood sugar level is over 300, check your infusion site and line to make sure it is not occluded. Bolus and retest one hour later to make sure your blood sugar is coming down. Do not eat until your blood sugar is under better control.

Insulin pumps "remember" when you took your last dose of insulin, and you will tell your pump how long the insulin tends to remain active in your body. (To do this, your doctor and pump coach will have you determine your basal rate, then take a dose of insulin and watch how long it has an impact on your blood sugar. For most people, regular insulin lasts for four to six hours in the body.) The pump should take into account your last dose of insulin and factor in any active insulin at the time of your second bolus to avoid "stacking" one dose of insulin on top of another, which can lead to hypoglycemia.

High-fat meals can present challenges in traditional boluses. Fat slows the absorption of carbohydrates. If you bolus before a high-fat meal, you may go low before the carbohydrates in the meal kick in. If you use a pump, you can actually give part of the insulin with the meal and extend the rest of the insulin over a period of hours after eating.

Some pumps have bolus settings for "normal" (all the insulin at once), "square" (the insulin spread out evenly over a fixed period of time), or "dual" (part of the insulin in the front and the rest spread out evenly over a fixed period of time). You have the choice of how you want to take the insulin each time you bolus.

Once your pump settings are established, be sure to write down all of your pump data on paper so that you won't have to start over with the programming if something should happen to your pump.

Living with the Pump

After going on an insulin pump, you will get used to the basic functions and begin to think of ways you can use your pump to obtain tighter blood sugar control. With most pumps you can program alternate basal rates, perhaps one for the days you work out and others for the days you don't plan to exercise.

You may create several different types of basal rates—one for hot days at the beach, when you will need less insulin, another for sick days, when you will need more insulin since blood sugar levels tend to rise. Some women learn that they need more insulin on the days before they begin their menstrual period, so they may develop a basal rate for those days. By using a pump, you can design a number of different basic basal rates so that you will have to make fewer corrections in your blood sugar throughout the day.

Troubleshooting High Blood Sugar

If you experience high blood sugar, you will need to troubleshoot the pump to make sure it is working properly. Common pump problems include the following:

- Empty reservoir: Most pumps send out an alarm when the insulin reservoir is running low, but sometimes people clear the alarms and forget to add insulin. Running out of insulin is like running out of gas: Your car still works, but it needs something to run on.

- Forgotten bolus: Believe it or not, you may actually sit down and eat and forget to bolus. You may not remember until you test your blood sugar two hours later and find it sky high. Pumps have bolus history functions that allow you to review the last bolus, so you can determine if you inadvertently missed a bolus.

- Low bolus: If you miscount the number of carbohydrates in a meal, you may under-bolus and your blood sugar will be high. If necessary, test your blood sugar again and give yourself a correction bolus.

- Sickness: As mentioned previously, illness can make your blood sugar run high. Put your sick plan into action. (For more information on sick plans, see Chapter 25.)

• Overuse of the same infusion site: If you repeatedly use the same area to place your infusion set, a fatty deposit may form and insulin absorption will be erratic and less effective. (This is the same problem that occurs if you inject insulin into the same area using needles.)

• Pump malfunction: Insulin pumps are machines, and machines break down. Most manufacturers have service programs that provide replacement pumps within 24 hours.

As a general rule, most doctors recommend that you give yourself a correction bolus if your blood sugar is too high. One hour later, retest. If your blood sugar has not gone down, replace the infusion set and re-bolus. In another hour, test again. If your blood sugar level has not dropped, use an injection and test your urine for ketones.

If you become an insulin pump user, you will find all kinds of tricks that will help you learn how to manage the pump to meet your lifestyle. While pump therapy isn't right for everyone, it does offer the opportunity for improved blood sugar control for many people with diabetes.

People with type 2 diabetes may or may not need insulin to control their condition. Those who do not need insulin typically do need to take oral diabetes medications, which are described in the following chapter.

CHAPTER 9
MEDICATION

When Bill learned he had type 2 diabetes, he willingly took the oral medication his doctor prescribed. "At first I thought I could take the pill and continue eating as I always had," he said. "When my blood sugar stayed high, I found out that I needed to change my eating habits as well. The treatment wasn't as easy as just popping a pill."

While oral diabetes medications can help people with type 2 diabetes bring their blood sugar numbers into their target zones, they can't make up for poor diet and exercise habits. "It's taken me a while, but I now try to follow the whole program."

Today, people like Bill with type 2 diabetes have several oral medications to choose from, but that was not always the case. Oral diabetic medications were discovered by accident during World War II. A French army doctor noticed that the soldiers he treated with sulfa antibiotics developed hypoglycemia, just as they would if they had taken too much insulin. He reasoned that the medication may have an effect on blood sugar levels. Other doctors found that taking sulfa drugs did, in fact, lower blood sugar levels, and a new use for this medication was developed.

In the years since this discovery, several oral medications have been developed for the treatment of type 2 diabetes. These drugs, known as oral hypoglycemic agents, play an essential role in the treatment of type 2 diabetes, although they do have unwanted side effects and they don't work for everyone.

Oral medications don't take the place of insulin. They are only effective in people who have a working pancreas. That means oral medications work for people with type 2 diabetes (because their bodies make insulin, but not enough), but they do not work in those with type 1 diabetes (because their bodies no longer produce any insulin). Remember, insulin can't be taken by mouth because it is destroyed by harsh stomach acids; it must be given by injection.

Oral diabetes medications work by increasing the amount of insulin released by the pancreas, increasing the sensitivity of the body to insulin, and decreasing the rate at which glucose is absorbed from the gastrointestinal tract.

Types of Oral Diabetes Medications

There are several types of oral diabetes medication, each of which works differently in the body.

- Sulfonylureas: These drugs, the first class of oral diabetes medications, encourage the pancreas to produce more insulin. The first-generation drugs tend to be less potent than the newer versions. Side effects include hypoglycemia, upset stomach, skin rash, itching, and weight gain.

First-generation drugs:
- Acetohexamide (Dymelor)
- Chlorpropamide (Diabinese)
- Tolbutamide (Orinase)
- Tolazamide (Tolinase)

Second-generation drugs:
- Glipizide (Glucotrol, Glucotrol XL)
- Glyburide (DiaBeta, Micronase, Glynase)
- Glimepiride (Amaryl)
- Gliclazide (Diamicron)

- Biguanides: These drugs help insulin move into the cells. They also inhibit the liver from releasing additional glucose, especially overnight. Biguanides should not be used by people with kidney problems or heart failure. Because it slows the release of glucose rather than making insulin more effective, there is little risk of hypoglycemia. Side effects include upset stomach and metallic taste in the mouth. It does not cause weight gain, and can contribute to weight loss, as well as lower cholesterol levels. It is usually the first-line medication used to treat type 2 diabetes.

Metformin (Glucophage, Glucophage XR, Riomet, Fortamet, and Glumetza)

- Thiazolidinediones: These drugs make insulin more effective. They also reduce the amount of glucose released by the liver and make cells more responsive to the effects of insulin. They should not be used by people with heart failure, due to an increased risk of heart attack and heart-related death. Side effects include high liver enzymes, liver failure, respiratory infection, headache, and fluid retention.

    Pioglitazone (Actos)
    Rosiglitazone (Avandia)

• Alpha-glucosidase inhibitors: These drugs slow the rise in blood sugar by blocking the enzymes that digest starches. Side effects include diarrhea, cramps, and gas.

    Acarbose (Precose and Glucobay)
    Miglitol (Glyset)

• Meglitinides: These drugs cause the pancreas to release more insulin when blood sugar is high. Side effects include hypoglycemia and upset stomach.

    Repaglinide (Prandin)
    Nateglinide (Starlix)

• Dipeptidyl peptidase IV inhibitors: These drugs increase insulin release and reduce the production of sugar by the liver when blood sugar levels are high. These drugs can be taken alone or in combination with other drugs.

    Januvia

- Combination therapy: Some drugs combine two medications in a single pill.

  Glucovance (a combination of glyburide and metformin)
  Metaglip (glipizide and metformin)
  Avandamet (metformin and Avandia)

Using Oral Diabetes Medications

The following tips may help you use oral diabetes medications safely and effectively to treat your type 2 diabetes:

- Take your medication every day. Oral diabetes medications should be taken regularly so that a steady amount of the drug remains in your system. These drugs are not intended to be used only when your blood sugar runs high. You will need to work with your doctor to determine the appropriate dose of any of the medications that will lower your blood sugar, but not put you at risk of hypoglycemia.

- If you have a history of allergic reactions to sulfa-based antibiotics, you may also be allergic to the sulfonylurea drugs. Discuss the issue with your doctor before taking the drugs.

- Some people find that oral diabetes medications become less effective over time as the pancreas grows weaker. Your doctor may be able to prescribe different drugs or combinations of drugs to help control blood sugar levels if they climb too high.

• Oral diabetes medications tend to be most effective in people who have had high blood sugar for less than 10 years and follow a healthy meal plan. They are less effective in people who are very thin.

It is important to remember that oral diabetes medications do not replace diet and exercise as the cornerstones of your treatment plan. You won't be able to indulge in high-sugar foods and sit on the couch, expecting to pop a pill and keep your blood sugar in check. A low-carbohydrate diet and regular exercise provide the foundation of good diabetic control. You will learn more about healthy eating in the following chapter.

CHAPTER 10
DIET

When Allan learned that he had type 2 diabetes, he feared that he would have to give up his obsession with hot dogs. Marilyn worried that she'd have to give up all forms of fast food, as well as her occasional indulgences of cakes and candies. Good news: While overeating any food isn't good for you whether or not you have diabetes, there is no need to give up any specific foods when you learn that you will have to watch your blood sugar. As you've no doubt heard before, moderation is key.

The diabetic diet is no different from the healthy eating plans recommended for people without diabetes. There is no need to eat special foods, give up favorite treats, or go hungry. Once you have been diagnosed with type 1 or type 2 diabetes, you will need to become more aware of the foods you eat and when you must eat them, but your healthy eating plan is not much different than the plan you should have been following all along.

If you have recently been diagnosed with diabetes, you may want to visit with a registered dietician who can help you plan your meals. This is especially important if you need to lose weight; if you have food allergies; or if you have high cholesterol, high triglycerides, high blood pressure, kidney disease, or any other medical issues that require you to follow a special diet.

There may be a registered dietician who works with your doctor. You may also want to contact the American Dietetic Association (www.eatright.org; 800-366-1655) or the American Association of Diabetes Educators (www.diabeteseducator.org; 800-832-6874) for referrals. Many registered dieticians are certified diabetes educators and can provide additional support in managing your overall care.

The Types of Nutrients

The food you eat is made up of one of three main types of nutrients: carbohydrates, proteins, and fats.

- **Carbohydrates** are the body's main source of energy. Fruits, vegetables, grains, and breads contain carbohydrates. Sugars—also honey, molasses, corn syrup, and other sweeteners—are also carbohydrates. The digestive system readily turns carbohydrates into glucose, which is released into the bloodstream. This rise in blood glucose is meant to fuel the cells of the body.

  Carbohydrates are most directly related to blood sugar levels. Sugar molecules are the building blocks of carbohydrates. When one or two sugar molecules are joined, they form a simple sugar. When long strands of sugar molecules are joined, they form complex carbohydrates, which don't taste sweet and must be digested in the stomach before being absorbed. Both simple and complex carbohydrates raise blood sugar levels.

• **Proteins** help to build and repair the tissue in the body. The body can convert proteins into glucose, but it takes longer. The digestive system breaks protein down into amino acids.

• **Fats** create energy reserves and help the cells of the body communicate. Fats are an essential part of a well-rounded diet. It is better to eat unsaturated fats (canola and olive oil, nuts and seeds) rather than saturated fats (butter, fatty meats, bacon, full-fat dairy products). Fats have twice as many calories per gram than carbohydrates or proteins, so you need to limit fat to control caloric intake.

Fats do not cause a rise in blood sugar, but they have an impact on blood sugar levels because they delay the time it takes for the blood sugar to rise from the carbohydrates eaten as part of the meal. In other words, if you had a roll with your dinner, the butter you put on the roll wouldn't increase your blood sugar, but it would cause your blood sugar to rise later than it would if you ate the roll without butter.

As you learn to eat within your diabetic meal plan, you will need to determine how much of the food you're eating consists of carbohydrates, proteins, and fats. This may sound difficult—and it may be tricky at first—but before long you'll be able to count the carbs in your meals without giving it a second thought.

Timing Is Everything

If you take insulin by injection, you will not only need to eat the right foods, but you will need to eat them at the right times. As noted earlier, insulin has peak times, and you will need to balance the insulin you take with the carbohydrates you eat.

You must schedule your meals and snacks based around the insulin peak times if you use injections. Try to create a routine and stick with it. You will need to

---

WHAT TO EAT

A balanced diet includes carbohydrates, proteins, and fats, although different amounts of each.

Carbohydrates

- Bread, cereal, rice, pasta, starchy vegetables (such as potatoes and corn), fruits.

- Eat 6 or more servings a day.

- A serving is 1/3 cup rice or pasta, 1/2 cup starchy vegetables, 1 slice of bread.

Fruits and Vegetables

- Eat 3 to 5 servings of vegetables and 2 to 4 servings of fruit.

---

work with your doctor and your dietician to design a meal schedule.

Real Sugar and Sugar Substitutes

For a long time, diabetics were told to avoid sugar. Experts now know that many different types of carbohydrates affect blood sugar levels and that sugar is not the only factor to worry about. Instead, you need to focus on the total amount of carbohydrate in a food.

- A serving is 1 cup raw or ½ cup cooked vegetables; 1 small piece or ½ cup canned fruit.

Protein

- Meat, poultry, seafood, fish, eggs, cheese, milk, yogurt, and peanut butter.

- Eat 4 to 6 servings of protein daily.

- A serving is 1 cup milk, 4 to 6 ounces meat, or 1 ounce cheese.

Fats and Sweets

- Fried foods, potato chips, candy, cakes.

- Limit these to the occasional treats; they should not be part of your basic meal plan.

There are two kinds of sweeteners: nutritive (which contain calories) and non-nutritive (which are calorie free). Table sugar or sucrose is the classic nutritive sweetener. Many foods contain corn syrup, dextrose, and maltose, all forms of nutritive sugar. Other more natural or less processed forms of sugar—honey, molasses, or unrefined sugar—have the same impact on blood sugar as refined sugar.

Fruit sugar or fructose causes blood sugar to rise less than refined sugar does, and when eaten in the form of a whole piece of fruit, the fiber in the fruit also helps offset the rise in blood sugar. If you're looking for a blast of

---

HOW SWEET IT IS

Non-Nutritive Sweeteners

- Saccharin (Sweet'n Low): 200 to 700 times sweeter than sucrose; can be used for cooking and baking

- Aspartame (NutraSweet, Equal): 160 to 220 times sweeter than sucrose; it may change flavor when heated

- Acesulfame-k (Sunette, Sweet One): 200 times sweeter than sucrose; can be used for cooking and baking

sweet that causes minimal impact on your blood sugar, opt for whole fresh fruit if you can.

Sugar substitutes such as saccharin, aspartame, and sucralose allow you to eat sweet-tasting foods without overdoing the carbs. Calorie-free sugar substitutes taste sweet but they don't cause a rise in blood sugar. Many foods containing these non-nutritive sweeteners are "free" (no carb) or low-carb foods and drinks.

Sugar alcohols are used to sweeten candy, gum, ice cream, baked goods, and other foods, as well as toothpaste, mouthwash, cough syrups, and other medications. The body absorbs sugar alcohol more slowly than other

- Sucralose (Splenda): 600 times sweeter than sucrose; can be used for cooking and baking

Nutritive Sweeteners

- Sucrose (table sugar, powdered sugar, brown sugar, molasses): classic sweetener

- Fructose (fruit sugar, high fructose corn syrup): can replace sucrose in baking; in large amounts it raises cholesterol

- Sugar alcohols (sorbitol, mannitol, xylitol, isomalt, lactitol, maltitol): 25 to 90 percent as sweet as sucrose; can have a laxative effect in large doses

sugars, so they cause a smaller rise in blood glucose. Many low-carb foods contain sugar alcohols.

Always check product labels. Many foods labeled "sugar free" still contain carbs, which will increase blood sugar levels. As a rule, avoid "fat-free" and "low-fat" products, which tend to have extra sugar added to make up for the missing fat. Likewise, check the labels on various "diet" or "sugar-free" products. Many of them contain almost the same number of total carbohydrates (so they will have the same impact on your blood sugar level), although they cost significantly more than traditional products.

If you have a sweet tooth, don't make yourself crazy by restricting all sweet foods. As long as your meal plan is reasonably well balanced, you can slip in the occasional indulgence without worrying too much about it, as long as you bolus for it. The problem isn't the periodic treat; it's your regular, day-to-day habit that you need to focus on. Stopping for ice cream or sticking your hand in the cookie jar every now and then won't hurt, and it can help you from feeling deprived.

Carb Counting and Exchange Lists

The key to knowing how much insulin to take is to know how much carbohydrate you need to cover with your bolus. The greater the number of carbohydrates you eat, the higher your blood sugar will go and the greater the amount of insulin you will need to keep your blood sugar in a healthy range. There are two main ways of determining carbohydrates—carb counting and exchange lists.

Carb Counting

Carb counting means just what it says: You count up the carbohydrates in the meal and use the information provided by your doctor (or programmed into your insulin pump) to determine how much insulin you need to take to cover the carbs. The only tricky part is learning to estimate the carbohydrate content of various foods. There are a number of guide books that can be helpful with this (many people with diabetes swear by the CalorieKing counter, available at most bookstores).

With experience, you will become much more comfortable estimating the carb count of individual foods and combination foods (such as a casserole). In addition, you will become comfortable making an honest assessment of your carbs, then testing your blood sugar in two hours; if you need more insulin, you can bolus again—and if you're a bit low and the insulin is still effective, you might need to eat a little something to prevent a low. Frankly, there is little substitute for experience: The more practice you get at counting carbs, the better you will be at doing it.

Some people with diabetes get distracted by the glycemic index of various foods. At this point, you shouldn't worry about the glycemic index, which assesses how quickly various carbohydrate-containing foods raise your blood sugar. The biggest problem with the glycemic index is that it only looks at one food at a time, and people usually eat a number of foods in a single meal. The proteins and fats eaten along with the carbohydrates can have a dramatic impact on the blood sugar rise. Other factors—including the ripeness of fruit, fiber content of food, and whether a food is cooked or raw—can have a significant impact on how a food changes blood sugar levels as well. In the future, doctors may create a new program that takes the glycemic index into account, but for now, if you're counting carbs, all you need to focus on is the carbohydrate content of the foods.

Exchange Lists

People who don't want to count carbohydrates may prefer to use exchange lists to choose the foods they should eat at each meal. These lists include foods that have approximately the same carbohydrate count, and nutritionists sometimes use them to help people eat a balanced diet.

Basically, exchange lists divide foods into six categories—starch, meat and meat substitutes, vegetables, fruits, milk, and fat. As part of your meal plan, you are supposed to eat a certain number of foods from each category at each meal, and you have the freedom to choose the foods you want from the lists. For example, if you have 2 meat exchanges they could be 2 ounces of roast beef, or 1 ounce of roast beef and ¼ cup of cottage cheese. In other words, the foods on the list are approximately equal in value and can be exchanged for one another. Your doctor or dietician will help you determine what exchanges should be included in your meal plan.

Food Exchanges

Starch List

One starch exchange equals 15 grams of carbohydrate, 3 grams of protein, 0 to 1 grams of fat, and 80 calories.

Bread

1	Bagel
2 slices	Bread, reduced calorie
1 slice	Bread, white, whole wheat, pumpernickel, rye
2	Bread sticks
$\frac{1}{2}$	English muffin
$\frac{1}{2}$	Hot dog bun or hamburger bun
$\frac{1}{2}$	Pita (6 inches across)
1 slice	Raisin bread, unfrosted
1	Roll, plain, small
1	Tortilla, corn (6 inches across)
1	Tortilla, flour (7 to 8 inches across)
1	Waffle ($4\frac{1}{2}$-inch square, reduced fat)

Cereals and Grains

$\frac{1}{2}$ cup	Bran cereals
$\frac{1}{2}$ cup	Bulgur
$\frac{1}{2}$ cup	Cereals
$\frac{3}{4}$ cup	Cereals, unsweetened
3 tablespoon	Cornmeal
$\frac{1}{3}$ cup	Couscous
3 tablespoon	Flour
$\frac{1}{4}$ cup	Granola, low-fat

½ cup	Grits
¼ cup	Muesli
½ cup	Oats
½ cup	Pasta
1½ cup	Puffed cereal
⅓ cup	Rice, white or brown
½ cup	Rice milk
½ cup	Sugar-frosted cereal
3 tablespoon	Wheat germ

Starchy Vegetables

⅓ cup	Baked beans
½ cup	Corn
1	Corn on cob, medium
1 cup	Mixed vegetables (corn, peas, or pasta)
½ cup	Peas, green
1	Potato, baked or boiled, small
½ cup	Potato, mashed
1 cup	Squash, winter
½ cup	Yam, sweet potato, plain

Crackers and Snacks

15 to 20	Chips, fat-free (tortilla, potato)
3	Graham crackers
24	Oyster crackers
3 cups	Popcorn (popped, low-fat)
¾ ounce	Pretzels
2	Rice cakes (4 inches)
6	Saltine crackers
2 to 5	Whole-wheat crackers, no fat

Beans, Peas, Lentils

½ cup	Beans and peas (garbanzo, pinto, kidney, black-eyed)
½ cup	Lentils
⅔ cup	Lima beans

Starchy Foods with Fat

1	Biscuit (2½ inches)
½ cup	Chow mein noodles
1	Corn bread (2-inch cube)
1 cup	Croutons
16 to 25	French fries
¼ cup	Granola
1	Muffin, small
2	Pancakes (4 inches)
3	Sandwich crackers (cheese or peanut butter)
⅓ cup	Stuffing (prepared)
2	Taco shells (6 inches)
4 to 6	Whole-wheat crackers (with fat)

Fruit

One fruit exchange equals 15 grams carbohydrate and 60 calories; includes skin, seeds, and rind.

Fruit

1	Apple, small
½ cup	Applesauce, unsweetened
4 rings	Apples, dried
8 halves	Apricots, dried
4 whole	Apricots, fresh
1	Banana, small

¾ cup	Blackberries
¾ cup	Blueberries
1 cup	Cantaloupe, small
12	Cherries, sweet, fresh
3	Dates
3 medium	Figs, fresh
½ cup	Fruit cocktail
½	Grapefruit, large
17	Grapes, small
1 cup	Honeydew melon
1	Kiwi
¾ cup	Mandarin oranges, canned
½ cup	Mango, small
1	Nectarine, small
1	Orange, small
1 cup	Papaya
1	Peach, medium, fresh
½ cup	Peaches, canned
½	Pear, large, fresh
½ cup	Pears, canned
½ cup	Pineapple, canned
¾ cup	Pineapple, fresh
2	Plums, small
3	Prunes, dried
2 tablespoon	Raisins
1 cup	Raspberries
1¼ cup	Strawberries
2	Tangerines, small
1¼ cup	Watermelon

Fruit Juice

$1/2$ cup	Apple juice or cider
$1/3$ cup	Cranberry juice cocktail
1 cup	Cranberry juice cocktail, reduced calorie
$1/3$ cup	Fruit juice blend
$1/3$ cup	Grape juice
$1/2$ cup	Grapefruit juice
$1/2$ cup	Orange juice
$1/2$ cup	Pineapple juice
$1/3$ cup	Prune juice

Milk

One milk exchange equals 12 grams carbohydrate and 8 grams of protein.

1 cup	Skim milk
1 cup	1% milk
1 cup	2% milk
1 cup	Whole milk
$1/2$ cup	Evaporated skim milk
$1/2$ cup	Evaporated whole milk
$1/3$ cup	Nonfat dry milk (dry)
1 cup	Non-fat or low-fat buttermilk
1 cup	Goat's milk
1 cup	Sweet acidophilus milk
1 cup	Non-fat or low-fat fruit yogurt (with aspartame)
$3/4$ cup	Plain low-fat yogurt
$3/4$ cup	Plain non-fat yogurt

Vegetable List

One vegetable exchange equals 5 grams of carbohydrate, 2 grams of protein, 0 grams of fat, and 25 calories.

NOTE: All portions are 1/2 cup cooked vegetables or 1 cup raw vegetables.

Artichokes, artichoke hearts, asparagus, beans, bean sprouts, beets, broccoli, Brussels sprouts, cabbage, carrots, cauliflower, celery, cucumber, eggplant, green onions, greens, leeks, mushrooms, okra, onions, pea pods, peppers, radishes, salad greens, spinach, squash, tomatoes, turnips, water chestnuts, zucchini.

Meats and Seafood

Very Lean

One very lean meat equals 0 grams carbohydrate, 7 grams protein, 0 to 1 gram fat, and 35 calories.

1 ounce	Chicken or turkey (white meat, no skin)
¼ cup	Egg substitute
2	Egg whites
1 ounce	Fat-free cheese
1 ounce	Fish (cod, flounder, haddock, halibut, trout, tuna; fresh or frozen)
1 ounce	Game meat (venison, buffalo, ostrich, duck; no skin)
¼ cup	Non-fat or low-fat cottage cheese
1 ounce	Shellfish (clams, crab, lobster, scallops, shrimp)

Lean

One lean meat exchange equals 0 grams carbohydrate, 7 grams protein, 3 grams fat, and 55 calories

¼ cup	4.5% cottage cheese
1 ounce	Cheese (3 grams of fat per ounce)
1 ounce	Chicken or turkey (dark meat, no skin)
1 ounce	Chicken or turkey (white meat, with skin)
2 tablespoon	Grated Parmesan
1 ounce	Lamb
1 ounce	Lean beef (USDA Select or Choice, trimmed of fat)
1 ounce	Lean pork
6	Oysters
1 ounce	Salmon, herring, tuna (in oil)
1 ounce	Veal

Average-Fat

Average-fat meat equals 0 grams carbohydrate, 7 grams protein, 5 grams fat, and 75 calories.

1 ounce	Cheese: Feta, mozzarella
1 ounce	Chicken or turkey (dark meat, with skin), ground turkey or chicken, fried chicken
1	Egg
1 ounce	Fried fish, any type
1 ounce	Ground beef, meatloaf, corned beef, ribs, Prime grade meats
1 ounce	Lamb (rib roast, ground)

1 ounce	Pork chops, cutlets
1 cup	Soy milk
½ cup	Tofu

High-Fat
High-fat meat equals 0 grams carbohydrate, 7 grams protein, 8 grams fat, and 100 calories.

3 slices	Bacon
1 ounce	Pork: Spareribs, ground pork, pork sausage
1 ounce	Processed sandwich meats with 8 grams fat (bologna, pimento loaf, etc.)
1 ounce	Regular cheese: American, Cheddar, Monterey Jack, Swiss

Fat
One fat exchange equals 5 grams fat and 45 calories.

Monounsaturated

6	Almonds, cashews, mixed nuts
1 ounce	Avocado
1 teaspoon	Oil: Canola, olive, peanut
8	Olives, large
2 teaspoon	Peanut butter
10	Peanuts

Polyunsaturated

1 tablespoon	Lower-fat margarine
1 teaspoon	Margarine, regular
1 tablespoon	Mayonnaise, low-fat

| 1 teaspoon | Mayonnaise, regular |
| 1 teaspoon | Oil: Corn, safflower, soybean |

Unsaturated

1 slice	Bacon
1 teaspoon	Butter
2 tablespoon	Coconut, sweetened, shredded
2 tablespoon	Cream, half and half
2 tablespoon	Cream cheese, reduced fat
1 tablespoon	Cream cheese, regular
3 tablespoon	Sour cream, reduced fat
2 tablespoon	Sour cream, regular

By using the exchange program, meals will contain approximately the same number of carbohydrates. You can discuss both methods of meal planning—counting carbohydrates and using food exchanges—with your doctor. Most people prefer counting carbohydrates, but both methods work if you're willing to follow them.

Smart Grocery Shopping

To be a careful grocery shopper, you will have to become a careful label reader. Here are some tips for becoming a savvy shopper:

• Don't get sidetracked by label claims of low-fat, fat-free, high-fiber, lite, sugar-free, or any other health benefit. The claim may be true, but that doesn't necessarily mean that the food is a good choice.

- Look at the carb count and serving size on the label so that you can decide if a given food is worth the carbs.

- Check the number of servings per container. Sometimes small packages contain more than one serving.

Eat Right
Good eating habits go beyond choosing the right foods:

- Start the day with breakfast. You'll be less likely to overeat later in the afternoon.

- Don't skip meals. Eating every few hours helps your body maintain steady blood sugar levels.

- Drink six to eight glasses of water a day. Water will keep you feeling full and it will help you digest the food you eat.

- Plan your meals. If you think about the foods you're going to get and plan ahead, you'll be more likely to have healthy foods on hand and more likely to skip the extra snacks during the day.

- Eat slowly. It takes at least 20 minutes for your brain to realize that your stomach is full. Give your body time to enjoy the food you're eating and to recognize the sensation of fullness before you've overeaten.

- Use your measuring cups, spoons, and scales to teach yourself how to estimate portion sizes accurately. As a rule of thumb, 1 cup of pasta is about the size of a clenched fist, ½ cup of vegetables is the size of half a tennis ball, and 1 ounce of cheese is about 1-inch square. The more often you measure your food, the more accurate your estimates will become.

- Eat a variety of foods. Mixing up your diet helps to ensure that you eat an adequate amount of different micronutrients.

- Don't keep tempting foods in the house. It's much harder to overindulge if your favorite foods aren't waiting for you on the kitchen shelf.

- Eat plant-based foods—that means fruits and vegetables. These foods tend to be nutrient dense and high fiber, so they will fill you up and nourish your body at the same time.

- If you slip up, don't fall. You will have days when you overeat and make poor food choices. Don't allow one unsuccessful day to become two. Instead, forgive yourself for your temporary lapse and continue to practice your healthy habits. Don't think you have to be perfect. Just make the best choices you can as often as you can.

- Ask for help. If you need help sticking to a healthy diet, ask your doctor for assistance. A dietician may be able to help you design a meal plan that includes the foods you miss in reasonable portions.

A Word About Alcohol

Alcohol presents unique challenges to the person with diabetes. Many people assume that alcohol is metabolized as sugar and contributes to high blood sugar, but this is not true. Alcohol is a toxin to the body, so the liver wants to get rid of it as soon as possible. If your blood sugar drops too low, the liver adds glucose to the blood. When the liver is busy working on removing the alcohol from the blood, it isn't tending to the fluctuations in your blood sugar, so your blood sugar can drop too low. That means that if you don't eat enough carbohydrates along with the alcohol, you may develop hypoglycemia. To make the situation more confusing and dangerous, the symptoms of low blood sugar can be confused with those of drunkenness, so it is more difficult to identify and treat episodes of hypoglycemia.

If you drink responsibly and want to include a single drink (that's 1½ ounces of liquor, 4 ounces of wine, or 12 ounces of beer) with your regular diet, you can probably do so safely. Check your blood sugar before, during, and after you consume any alcohol. Alcohol can lower your blood sugar for 8 to 12 hours after your last drink.

As a diabetic, you cannot safely drink to excess, even if you consume carbohydrates. If you have difficulty limiting your alcohol intake, talk to your doctor about your concerns. Pregnant women, people with a history of alcohol abuse, and people with diabetic complications should avoid all alcohol. Also skip the drink if you have just exercised vigorously, if you are taking prescription or over-the-counter medications that react with alcohol, or if you have an empty stomach. In addition, keep in mind that alcohol can worsen diabetic complications, including nerve damage, eye disease, and high blood pressure.

Reaching a Healthy Weight

According to the National Institutes of Health, more than half of all Americans are overweight or obese. The extra pounds put you at increased risk of heart disease, high blood pressure, stroke, arthritis, and diabetes, among other problems.

Weight loss is especially important for people with type 2 diabetes who are obese. If you have type 2 diabetes and you lose weight and exercise regularly, you may be able to avoid the need for oral diabetes medications or insulin. Weight loss is essential because the more overweight you are, the more resistance you have to your insulin. That means a specific amount of insulin doesn't work as well as it should. Your pancreas will then have to work harder to provide still more insulin. Eventually the pancreas can't keep up with the demand, and your blood sugar begins to climb.

The key to losing weight is to consume fewer calories than your body requires each day. So what's that magic number? To estimate the calories you need to stay the weight you are now, calculate 10 calories per pound of body weight, plus:

- 20 % for a sedentary lifestyle
- 33 % for light physical activity daily
- 50 % for moderate physical activity daily
- 75 % for a very active lifestyle

For example, if you weigh 150 pounds and live a moderately active life, the calories you need to remain the same weight would be $150 \times 10 = 1,500$, plus 750 $(1,500 \times .50)$ or 2,250 calories. This is a very crude measure, but it gives you a rough approximation of the calories you would need to maintain your body weight.

To lose weight, you need to eat fewer calories than you consume. If your daily caloric requirement was 2,250 and you cut back 500 calories a day, you could consume about 1,750 a day and lose about a pound a week. (One pound equals about 3,500 calories.)

You can either work with a dietician or design your own food plan that contains the appropriate number of daily calories. Don't try to rush things and lose too much weight too fast or you'll slow your metabolism and invariably become frustrated and throw in the towel. The secret to success is gradual weight loss. Even a modest weight loss can go a long way toward improving your blood sugar control and reducing your risk of health problems.

Celiac Disease

A disproportionate number of people with type 1 diabetes also suffer from celiac disease, a digestive disorder that interferes with the body's ability to tolerate the gluten found in wheat, oats, barley, and rye.

Like type 1 diabetes, celiac is an autoimmune disease. When the body is exposed to gluten, the immune system triggers an inflammatory process in the small intestine and it attacks the villi, the hairlike projections in the small intestine that absorb nutrients from food. If the condition is untreated, the small intestine cannot absorb food and nutrients, leading to vitamin deficiencies, malnutrition, osteoporosis, neurological disorders, and cancer.

Celiac disease was once thought to be rare, but it is now being called one of the most underdiagnosed common diseases in the United States. About 1 out of 10 people with type 1 diabetes in the U.S. is affected by celiac disease compared with an estimated 1 out of 100 in the general population. The incidence of celiac disease among people, particularly children with type 1 diabetes, has led an increasing number of health-care professionals and parents to call for routine screening of all people with type 1 diabetes to look for the presence of antibodies for celiac disease.

The onset of celiac disease typically occurs in childhood at three to five years of age and in adulthood during the thirties and forties. Symptoms of celiac disease include stomachaches and digestive problems after eating, anemia, fatigue, and depression. The condition can also cause failure to grow and thrive, especially in babies. However, about half of all people diagnosed with celiac do not have any symptoms at all.

My daughter was screened for celiac one year after her initial diagnosis. She had antibodies indicating the presence of the disease, and a biopsy of her small intestine confirmed the diagnosis. She never complained of any symptoms. For a while, my husband and I wondered whether we needed to go to the trouble of having the biopsy, but the doctor convinced us that it was important because the diet is lifelong and difficult to live with and since she didn't have any symptoms, she would be tempted to challenge the diagnosis when she got older. The biopsy confirmed the diagnosis.

Some people experience symptoms of celiac disease for years without understanding the cause of their discomfort. When they are diagnosed with the disease, they feel relieved because they now understand what is happening in their bodies and what can be done to ease the pain.

Bennett suffered from stomachaches and cramping for almost 10 years before the doctor treating her type 1 diabetes suggested that she be tested for celiac disease. When the results came back positive, the 18-year-old felt distressed that she had another autoimmune disease.

"I didn't want to have another disease to worry about, but at least this one didn't require needles," Bennett said. "I feel better than I ever have before, so that makes it worth giving up some foods I like."

In addition to eating a balanced diet and counting carbohydrates, many people with diabetes benefit from taking certain nutritional supplements to make up for deficiencies in their diets. The following chapter discusses key nutritional supplements that can help enhance blood sugar control.

CHAPTER 11
NUTRITIONAL SUPPLEMENTS

His friends and family call him the Medicine Man. Every morning Dan takes his diabetes medication, as well as a multivitamin, chromium, calcium, and several other vitamin and mineral supplements. "I call this my supplemental insurance plan," says the 62-year-old type 2 diabetic. "These supplements help ensure that my blood sugar numbers are low."

While insulin is the mainline drug for type 1 diabetics and oral medication helps those with type 2, there is evidence that people with both forms of diabetes can benefit from some over-the-counter nutritional supplements. Of course, taking supplements can't make up for poor eating and exercise habits, but they can help many people improve their blood sugar control.

Supplement manufacturers advertise scores of products that claim to support people with diabetes, but this chapter will focus on a few key supplements which have clinical research to back up the claims.

Most Helpful Supplements

- **Chromium** is an essential trace mineral that improves glucose tolerance, in addition to assisting with the synthesis of cholesterol, fats, and proteins. Chromium makes insulin about 10 times more efficient at processing sugar, so less insulin is needed to do the job.

  About 90 percent of the population does not get enough chromium from food. In addition, a high-sugar diet can increase the excretion of chromium, contributing to diabetes. Some experts believe chromium deficiency may contribute to the surge in type 2 diabetes in the United States.

  Nearly 20 controlled studies have demonstrated a positive effect from chromium in the treatment of diabetes. Most of the studies were performed on people with type 2 diabetes.

  Take 200 micrograms of chromium daily.

  Chromium can also be found in brewer's yeast, wheat germ, corn oil, whole grain cereals, meats, cheese, bran, liver, kidney, oysters, molasses, potatoes with the skin on, peanuts, and peanut butter. (Refining and processing foods dramatically reduces chromium levels in foods.)

- **Fenugreek** is a member of the legume family and is one of the world's oldest medicinal herbs. In many parts of the world it is used as a food and a spice, as well as for medicinal purposes. The seeds of the fenugreek plant contain alkaloids, which reduce the amount of sugar in the urine and improve glucose tolerance.

Studies have shown that this herb can reduce urine sugar levels by up to 50 percent. Researchers have used 15 to 100 grams of fenugreek powder daily to treat people with type 2 diabetes.

> Fenugreek is available in commercially prepared supplements, but do not take fenugreek for blood sugar control without your doctor's guidance.

> Fenugreek is a spice found in many curry preparations.

- **Biotin**, also known as vitamin B$_7$ and vitamin H, is a member of the B vitamin family. It enhances insulin sensitivity and improves the utilization of blood sugar, in addition to facilitating the use of the other B vitamins. The blood sugar response is thought to be the result of an increase in the activity of the enzyme glucokinase, which is involved in the utilization of blood sugar by the liver.

  In one study, 8 milligrams of biotin twice daily resulted in significant lowering of fasting blood sugar levels and improved blood sugar control in type 1 diabetics. In a study of type 2 diabetics, similar effects were noted with 9 milligrams of biotin daily.

Take 9 to 16 milligrams daily, under a doctor's supervision. (If you take biotin, you may need to adjust the dosage of your insulin or oral diabetes medications.)

Biotin can also be found in soy, whole grains, egg yolks, almonds, walnuts, oatmeal, mushrooms, broccoli, bananas, peanuts, liver, kidney, milk, legumes, sunflower seeds, and nutritional yeast.

• **Magnesium** is involved in a number of crucial bodily functions, from the creation of bone to the beating of the heart and the balance of sugar in the bloodstream. Many diabetics have a deficiency in magnesium; supplements (even at low doses) tend to minimize complications related to diabetes. Poor blood sugar control can lead to magnesium deficiency and insulin insensitivity. In people with an established magnesium deficiency, magnesium supplements can help improve blood sugar control.

Take 300 to 400 milligrams of magnesium chloride daily.

Magnesium is found in nuts, whole grains, wheat bran, dark green vegetables, brown rice, garlic, apples, bananas, apricots, beans, dairy products, meat, fish, oysters, and scallops.

• **Manganese** is a mineral that is involved with many enzyme reactions, including those responsible for

THE COMPLETE GUIDE TO LIVING WELL WITH DIABETES 143

controlling blood sugar levels. It also assists in blood clotting, the production of energy from food, and the synthesis of protein. Manganese levels in diabetics tend to be about half the levels found in people without diabetes.

Take 30 milligrams of manganese daily.

Manganese is found in nuts, wheat bran, avocados, leafy green vegetables, pineapple, dried fruits, coffee, tea, and seeds.

Other Helpful Supplements

• **Inositol** is a B vitamin supplement that the body uses to produce lecithin and to transfer fats from the liver to the cells in the body. It also helps maintain normal nerve function. Diabetic neuropathy is one of the most common complications of longterm diabetes. Much of the decrease in nerve function is due to the loss of inositol from the nerve cells.

Take 500 milligrams of inositol twice daily.

Inositol is found in dried beans, chickpeas, lentils, cantaloupe, nuts, citrus, whole grain products, and wheat germ.

• **Coenzyme Q-10** is a vitaminlike substance sometimes referred to as ubiquinone. It is found in almost every cell of the body, but it is concentrated in the mitochondria of cells, where energy is produced. Coenzyme Q-10 helps transform food into energy. It is also a potent antioxidant.

Take 120 milligrams of Coenzyme Q-10 daily. (To optimize the benefits and absorption of Coenzyme Q-10, take the supplement with a little fat, such as peanut butter.)

• **Vitamin B$_6$** (pyridoxine) is one of the water-soluble B-complex vitamins. Its main functions in the body are to help release energy from food, aid in the proper functioning of more than 60 enzymes, and promote a healthy immune system. It also improves glucose tolerance. People with diabetic neuropathy have been shown to be deficient in vitamin B^6 and to benefit from supplementation.

Take 200 milligrams of vitamin B$_6$ daily.

Vitamin B$_6$ is also found in meats, fish, nuts, legumes, bananas, brown rice, avocados, whole grains, lentils, corn, eggs, fortified cereals, spinach, potatoes, soybeans, liver, kidney, poultry, oatmeal, and prunes.

• **Vitamin C**, a water-soluble vitamin, is a powerful antioxidant and immune system enhancer. It is transported into the cells using insulin. Many diabetics develop vitamin C deficiencies in the cells, even if they consume enough in their diets. Failure to address the problem with additional supplementation can lead to health problems, including poor wound healing, high cholesterol levels, and a depressed immune system.

Take 1,000 to 3,000 milligrams of vitamin C daily.

Vitamin C is found in citrus fruits, red bell peppers, kale, kiwi, broccoli, Brussels sprouts, cauliflower, strawberries, red cabbage, cantaloupe, rose hips, spinach, tomatoes, green peppers, parsley, dark green leafy vegetables, and potatoes.

• **Vitamin E** is a fat-soluble vitamin that has strong antioxidant properties. It improves glucose tolerance and helps the body maintain normal blood sugar levels. Vitamin E also plays a major role in maintaining proper functioning of the muscles and nerves.

Take 400 IU of vitamin E daily.

Vitamin E is found in asparagus, avocados, whole grain cereals, dark green leafy vegetables, poultry, eggs, seafood, seeds, nuts, wheat germ, and various oils (sunflower, almond, wheat germ, and hazelnut).

• **Garlic** helps lower blood sugar levels. It is one of the oldest and most commonly used medicinal plants. It contains sulfur compounds, which give it antibiotic properties.

> Eat three to six cloves of garlic daily, or use a commercially prepared product.

• **Ginseng** has long been used to treat diabetes. Double-blind studies have shown that ginseng can improve glucose control and increase energy among people with type 2 diabetes.

Ginseng is available in several species: Siberian ginseng, American ginseng, Chinese or Korean ginseng, and Japanese ginseng. The most common form is Chinese ginseng.

> Commercial products are available; follow package directions.

• **Soluble fiber** has been shown to help keep blood sugar under control. Fiber may also help prevent the development of type 2 diabetes; in a large-scale study of nurses in the United States, women who consumed the most whole-grain foods in their diets were nearly 40 percent less likely to develop diabetes than those who consumed the least.

> To help control sugar levels, eat a diet rich in beans and other foods high in soluble fiber. The type of bean doesn't matter, so enjoy red, white, and navy beans; lentils; garbanzos; and pinto beans.

Soluble fiber supplements are also available; follow package directions.

It is essential that your doctor have a comprehensive idea of all medications—both prescription and over-the-counter—that you take on a regular basis. Be sure to let your doctor know of all supplements you may be taking and at what doses.

While maintaining a healthy and balanced diet and taking appropriate nutritional supplements will help you control your diabetes, exercise also plays a critical role. The importance of exercise and ways to achieve your exercise goals will be discussed in the following chapter.

CHAPTER 12
EXERCISE

James discovered that he had type 2 diabetes when he was in his fifties. He didn't want to take insulin, so he told his doctor that he would walk for one hour after each meal. For more than 20 years—in rain, snow, and oppressive heat—he faithfully walked three times a day, a total of 21 miles a week. He never took insulin, and his blood sugar was in the normal range.

Exercise plays an essential role in diabetes management. Exercise improves blood sugar control, helps with weight control, reduces risk of heart disease, lowers blood pressure, minimizes the need for insulin and oral diabetes medication—not to mention the fact that you will look and feel marvelous. No matter what your age or level of fitness, exercise can improve your physical and emotional health and reduce your risk of serious illness.

You don't have to spend hours in the gym to enjoy these benefits of exercise. Recent studies have shown that as little as 30 minutes a day of light physical activity will offer significant health benefits. Yes, that's physical activity, not hard-core exercise. The time you spend strolling the neighborhood, walking the dog, climbing the stairs, and mowing the lawn counts toward your goal. Other studies have shown that you don't even have to do your 30 minutes of activity all at once, as long as you total a half hour during the course of the day.

Of course, before you start an exercise program, you should talk to your doctor if:

- You're planning a dramatic change in your activity level.

- You're over age 50.

- You're obese.

- You're a smoker.

- You have a history of heart disease.

- You're taking insulin and need to change your medication on exercise days.

- You have complications of diabetes, such as neuropathy (see Chapter 18) or retinopathy (see Chapter 16).

You should start any exercise program slowly and gradually build up the intensity of your workouts. Try to choose activities that you enjoy, and vary your exercise routine so you don't get bored. If you used to enjoy a certain activity in the past, try to reconnect with your inner athlete. Dig out the tennis racket from the hall closet and buy a new tin of balls, or put on your walking shoes and take the dog out for a long walk.

Some people like to work out alone; others prefer company. Some people like to exercise at home; others prefer the social atmosphere of a gym. There is no right or wrong way to build exercise into your daily routine, as long as you make a commitment to regular movement for at least 30 minutes three or four times a week.

Designing a Workout Plan

A well-rounded exercise program strives to build aerobic fitness, muscle strength, and flexibility. While you won't necessarily do all types of exercise during every workout, your weekly routine should include all three types of exercise.

Aerobic Fitness

If you don't exercise regularly, you have almost certainly lost aerobic power over the years, and you probably know it. Without exercise you will steadily lose aerobic conditioning. By age 65, the average person's aerobic capacity has dropped by about 40 percent, compared to the relatively fit days of young adulthood.

The term "aerobic" means "using oxygen." During aerobic exercise, your heart and lungs work harder than normal to provide your muscles with the oxygen they demand, and you must breathe heavily and steadily to meet your body's increased need for oxygen. During anaerobic exercise, your heart and lungs cannot meet your body's oxygen demands for longer than a short burst of activity, and you are left gasping for breath, even if you're in great shape. In other words, jogging around the track is aerobic exercise, and sprinting 50 yards is anaerobic exercise.

To improve your level of aerobic fitness and strengthen your heart and lungs, you need to perform some type of aerobic exercise, such as walking, jogging, bicycling, swimming, cross-country skiing, aerobic dancing, or rope skipping. These activities involve the rhythmic, repeated use of the major muscle groups. When done regularly, aerobic activities improve the efficiency of the heart, lungs, and muscles, and increase their ability to do work.

When assessing the intensity of your exercise plan, you can use your heart rate or pulse to determine how hard you're working. Your maximal heart rate is considered 220 minus your age. If you are 50 years old, for example, your maximum heart rate would be 170 beats per minute (220 minus 50).

Low-intensity exercise would be 20 minutes of activity at a heart rate equal to about 60 percent of your maximum heart rate. Very high intensity exercise would be 60 minutes of activity at a heart rate equal to about 80 percent of your maximum. Most people want to work out at an intermediate intensity (50 to 70 percent of maximum) for 20 to 30 minutes, at least three times a week.

If you aren't enthusiastic about exercise, you'll be pleased to know that even low-intensity exercise provides some health benefits. As you might imagine, some exercise is better than none. Try to start with a plan that is reasonable, and add intensity or duration to your workout over time. If you start out with an overly ambitious plan, you're more likely to become frustrated and quit. Your goal is to create a lifetime fitness plan that you can modify—but not abandon—as the years go by.

Be sure to warm up for 5 to 10 minutes by doing light calisthenics before your aerobic workout. You might also go through the motions of the main workout at a slower pace as a warm-up.

Also remember to cool down. After your workout, walk slowly for 3 to 5 minutes, or until your heart rate returns to just 10 or 15 beats above the resting rate. (The less fit you are, the more time you'll need for a cool down.) Stopping suddenly can cause the blood to pool in the legs, reducing blood pressure and possibly causing fainting.

Muscle Strength

Weight lifting and isometric exercises can be used to maintain strong muscles for a lifetime. Without strength training, you will lose muscle mass and strength: The average American loses 10 to 20 percent of muscle strength between the ages of 20 and 50, and then another 25 to 30 percent between 50 and 70. Strength training helps stave off these changes in the body.

In addition, strength training raises the basal metabolic rate, or the number of calories the body burns at rest. The more muscle you have, the higher your metabolic rate, the more calories you burn, and the easier it is to fight flab. Studies have shown that people who maintain their aerobic fitness still lose muscle mass—about one pound of muscle every two years after age 20—if they don't diversify their workouts to include strength training.

Flexibility

Flexibility is a critical part of fitness but one that is often overlooked. Flexibility involves more than touching your toes; it involves maintaining the range of motion in your joints. The only way to preserve your flexibility is to perform stretching exercises regularly.

As little as 10 minutes of stretching every other day can help to prevent stiffness and loss of flexibility. Don't stretch "cold" muscles. Instead, stretch 2 or 3 minutes into your warm-up, just after you have broken a sweat. To build flexibility, bend or flex until you feel tension or slight discomfort—but not pain—and hold each stretch for 20 to 60 seconds. Do not hold your breath, and do not bounce or pulse, which can tear the connective tissue in the joints.

Exercise and Blood Sugar

Exercise can trigger unpredictable changes in blood sugar. While exercise typically causes blood sugar to drop, in some circumstances it can actually cause a surge in glucose levels. In other words, exercise can cause hypoglycemia or hyperglycemia, depending on the circumstances.

Keep the following rules in mind:

Do not exercise if your blood sugar is over 250. If your blood sugar is high, your body may not have enough insulin on board to use the sugar in the blood. As described in Chapter 1, at these times, the cells are actually starved for glucose while excess sugar is concentrated in the blood. If you exercise when your body is in this state, rather than using the sugar in your blood, your liver releases extra glucose in a misguided attempt to feed the cells. In this situation, your blood sugar will go up if you exercise.

For some people, this unexpected reaction occurs when the blood sugar is 180, for others not until the blood sugar is over 250 or 300. You will have to experience this situation for yourself to determine how your body reacts to this stress, but, as a general rule, avoid exercise if your blood sugar is over 250.

Eat a meal one or two hours before exercising. You want your body to have begun the process of digestion and to have the carbohydrates from the meal available to the body during exercise.

Take insulin more than one hour before exercise. Taking insulin before exercise can speed its impact and cause hypoglycemia, especially if the insulin is injected into the muscles being exercised.

Keep an easy-to-digest source of carbohydrates (such as juice or non-chocolate candies) with you during exercise. You will probably need to consume extra carbohydrates after approximately every 30 minutes of moderate exercise.

After your workout, allow yourself to consume a little more food (or decrease your insulin or oral medication) during 12 to 24 hours after exercise since your metabolism will be higher and your body will be taking glucose from your bloodstream to replenish the glucose taken from the muscles during exercise.

This post-exercise drop in blood sugar can lead to serious hypoglycemia if you're not careful. My daughter joined the family in about two hours of vigorous cross-country skiing when the temperature was in the low 30s. I tested her blood sugar every 20 or 30 minutes and gave her 5 to 10 Skittles candies every 15 minutes or so. Her blood sugar was perfect—120 flat—during the entire afternoon.

Overnight, however, I checked her blood sugar every hour until 5 A.M. and gave her a total of seven juice boxes throughout the night. Again, her blood sugar remained on target and relatively flat, but only because I tanked her up with juice every hour. I knew she had worked hard, but I honestly didn't expect to have to give her more than 100 grams of carbohydrates through the night. I now expect that any time she does more than one hour of vigorous exercise, I will probably send her to bed with a blood sugar level of at least 180, and then check her at least twice in the night to make sure her levels don't creep up or down.

Everyone is different, so you will have to find out for yourself how your body responds to exercise. The key is to test your blood sugar every 20 or 30 minutes during exercise and to test every few hours in the 24 hours after exercise to determine if you experience hypoglycemia in the post-exercise period.

Exercise Caution

People with diabetes need to pay attention to their unique challenges.

Take care of your feet. Always wear appropriate footwear, and check your feet after working out. Treat blisters immediately. If necessary, consult a podiatrist.

Avoid exercise in extreme hot or cold. Extreme temperatures can affect blood sugar levels, making you more susceptible to hypoglycemia. If you do work out in hot or cold weather, be sure to check your blood sugar often.

Always wear a diabetes bracelet or necklace when exercising outside of your home. If you experience hypoglycemia and have a medical problem, it is essential that those around you realize that you have diabetes.

If you have advanced complications, talk to your doctor before starting any exercise plan. For example, people with advanced retinopathy, or multiple bleeds in their eyes, should be very careful about heavy lifting and intense exercise, which can make the situation worse.

Exercise can help control blood sugar levels during pregnancy. Talk to your doctor about the appropriate intensity of exercise based on your pre-pregnancy activity level and symptoms. Avoid exercises that raise the core body temperature above 100 degrees, such as exercising in high heat, taking a sauna, or soaking in a hot tub after your workout. If you didn't work out much before conception, you probably want to limit yourself to low-intensity exercise, based on your doctor's recommendations.

Once you start exercising, keep at it. Consistency counts. If you miss a few days of exercise, don't feel guilty and throw in the towel. Instead, just get back to it, but don't try to make up for lost time by increasing the intensity of your workout. In fact, if you skip exercise for one week, cut back on the intensity of your workout and gradually build up again. You start to lose aerobic conditioning and strength if you sit it out for as little as one week.

Regular exercise can go a long way toward improving your overall health and maintaining good blood sugar levels. While blood sugar control is always important, it is especially critical when a woman is pregnant. The following chapter explains how to control diabetes during pregnancy to ensure both a healthy baby and a healthy mother.

CHAPTER 13
DIABETES AND PREGNANCY

Louise could not have been more thrilled to learn that she was pregnant. A fitness instructor, she prided herself on staying in shape, and being pregnant only strengthened her resolve to continue to exercise and eat right—not just for herself but for her baby as well. That's why she was devastated during the sixth month of her pregnancy to learn that she had gestational diabetes.

"It really never occurred to me that I would develop diabetes," Louise said. "My pregnancy was normal and I was doing everything right." As Louise learned, diabetes—including gestational diabetes—isn't a punishment for people who don't take care of themselves.

Louise continued to do everything right: She learned how to inject insulin and she monitored her blood sugar carefully throughout the rest of her pregnancy. Her daughter was born full term and in perfect health.

Every pregnancy is stressful, but pregnancy can be particularly stressful when the mother has diabetes. It's always important to control your blood sugar levels, but the nine months you are pregnant are arguably the most critical months to manage your diabetes, both for your health and the health of your unborn child.

There are two types of diabetes that affect pregnant women:

- Gestational diabetes describes a previously non-diabetic woman who develops diabetes during her pregnancy.

- Pregestational diabetes refers to a woman with preexisting diabetes who becomes pregnant.

Women with gestational or pregestational diabetes must maintain excellent blood sugar control to avoid serious complications with the pregnancy.

Gestational Diabetes

Gestational diabetes usually appears sometime during the third trimester, when the fetus is growing larger and the pancreas is under greater strain. Most obstetricians screen for gestational diabetes by testing for sugar in urine samples given at regular well-baby appointments, and by performing a glucose challenge sometime during the 24th to 28th weeks of pregnancy. The pregnancy glucose challenge involves consuming 50 grams of carbohydrate and drawing a blood sample one hour later. If the blood sugar is elevated one hour after consuming the sugar, the doctor will probably recommend a full glucose challenge test. (For more information on glucose testing, see Chapter 2.)

An estimated 2 to 5 percent of pregnant American women develop gestational diabetes. The hormones produced by the placenta interfere with insulin, creating insulin resistance. If the pancreas cannot keep up with the increased demand for insulin, the woman develops gestational diabetes. When the hormone levels return to normal after the baby is delivered, the diabetes disappears in three out of four women. Having gestational diseases does, however, indicate that the pancreas does not respond well to stress. Women with gestational diabetes are at increased risk of developing type 2 diabetes later in life. If you have gestational diabetes, you should make a special effort to maintain a healthy weight, exercise regularly, and eat right to minimize the risk factors that you can control.

Gestational diabetes increases the risk of miscarriage and complications with the baby. The oral medications often used to treat type 2 diabetes cannot be used due to the risk to the developing fetus, so the mother must test blood sugar regularly, and inject insulin, if necessary.

Pregestational Diabetes

If you have type 1 diabetes, you should discuss your plans with your doctor before conceiving a child. While many women successfully deliver healthy babies without complications, some women with pregestational diabetes may face serious issues with pregnancy. As a general rule, the more complications you have prior to conception, the greater the likelihood that you will have a difficult pregnancy. For example, if your kidneys have been damaged due to the diabetes, you're more likely to develop hypertension and toxemia while pregnant.

For the most part, if you develop long-term complications while pregnant, the chances are good that those symptoms will reverse when the baby is delivered. However, if you already have serious long-term complications, those problems may become worse and you may not rebound as easily. Many doctors do not recommend that women with serious long-term diabetic complications consider pregnancy. If you are in good overall health aside from the diabetes, and you're willing to redouble your efforts to maintain good blood sugar levels, then pregnancy may be an option for you.

Having a Healthy Baby

No woman can be guaranteed a normal, successful pregnancy. In fact, about 16 percent of pregnancies among non-diabetic women end in miscarriage. (Many of these miscarriages occur before the woman realizes she is pregnant, and often these fetuses suffer from a terminal abnormality.) Among women with gestational diabetes, the miscarriage rate is the same as in women without diabetes.

Another major concern is birth defects, both major and minor. These are known as congenital anomalies. Minor anomalies include webbed toes, skin discolorations, and problems that can be corrected easily and do not have long-term health consequences. Major anomalies include spina bifida, heart problems, and other issues that threaten the baby's health.

The risk of major anomalies is about 2 to 3 percent in a woman without diabetes, but it jumps to 7 to 13 percent in those who have poorly controlled gestational diabetes. With well-controlled diabetes, that rate drops back to 1 to 5 percent.

Women with diabetes also run the risk of macrosomia, the medical term for a large, fat baby. As a rule, that means a baby more than 10 pounds, only it depends in part on the size of the parents. The problem occurs because the mother's blood glucose passes to the baby, but her insulin does not. The baby's pancreas produces lots of insulin and the baby's blood sugar is high, so the baby grows excessively large. If the mother's blood sugar is normal, the baby remains normal body weight.

Large babies can present challenges with delivery, especially for a small mother. Labor may be longer and more difficult, and sometimes a cesarean section is necessary.

In addition, babies born to diabetic mothers with poor control tend to have more problems during the first few weeks of life. The two most common problems are neonatal hypoglycemia and complications caused by premature birth.

Because the baby's pancreas has been working overtime pumping out large amounts of insulin while in the womb, it may produce too much insulin—causing hypoglycemia or low blood sugar—before the baby adjusts to its own insulin demands. This problem can be avoided if the mother has good control of her diabetes, and, even if the condition does occur, it can be controlled in the hospital provided the health-care staff is watching for it.

Large babies born to diabetic mothers may appear to be fully developed, but many are premature. The baby may be large, but the organs could still be underdeveloped. Depending on the severity of the condition, this condition may require medical attention, just as other premature babies require special care.

The Challenge of Blood Sugar Control During Pregnancy

Wild fluctuations in hormone levels occur during pregnancy, which can make it extraordinarily difficult to

maintain good blood sugar control, even if you are dili-
gent. If you take insulin, you can expect a significant increase in your insulin requirements, especially during the
third trimester. Many women also experience diabetic
complications, such as retinopathy or hypertension, but
these symptoms are usually temporary and disappear after the baby is born.

Ideally, a pregnant diabetic woman should strive for
the same blood sugar levels as a pregnant non-diabetic
woman. In numerical terms, that would be about 60 to 90
before meals and at bedtime, and below 140 two hours
after eating.

If you're dealing with gestational diabetes or type 2 diabetes, you may be able to reach those targets because
your pancreas is still doing most of the work. By controlling your diet and exercise, you may be able to ease the
burden on your pancreas enough to keep your blood sugars in the optimal zone.

If you have type 1 diabetes, it will be more challenging
for you to maintain optimal blood sugar levels. Let's face
it, it was incredibly difficult before conception, and your
body is under even more stress now. Brief elevations in
blood sugar aren't likely to cause serious problems, but
you will need to be attentive to your blood sugar levels at
all times. Do the best you can and work with your endocrinologist and obstetrician and the odds are excellent that
you can enjoy a successful pregnancy if you have good
control and few long-term complications.

You must also watch for ketones during your pregnancy. Ketones may be present if you aren't eating enough
calories or if your blood sugar is too high because you're

not getting enough insulin (ketoacidosis). Ketoacidosis puts the pregnancy at serious risk of miscarriage.

Check your urine for ketones daily. (See Chapter 5 for information on ketone testing.) If you have ketones and your blood sugar is normal, you need to consume more calories daily to keep up with your body's increased caloric needs during pregnancy. If you're spilling ketones in your urine and you have high blood sugar numbers, you must take steps to lower your blood sugar immediately by taking additional insulin.

Special Concerns of Diabetic Mothers

Expectant mothers with diabetes face a number of unique challenges that may require a different approach to managing their pregnancies.

Test your blood sugar more often. During pregnancy, your goal is tight blood sugar control. To avoid highs or lows, you will need to test even more often than usual. Most doctors recommend testing before each meal, two hours after each meal, before bed, at 2 A.M., and before driving. The tighter your control, the more likely you are to experience low blood sugar, so be sure to keep a reliable source of sugar with you at all times.

Redefine high. When you are pregnant, you should consider a blood sugar level of 180 to 200 too high. Pregnant women can enter ketoacidosis with blood sugars not much higher than 200. If you recognize a pattern in your highs—you're running high in the mornings when you wake up, for example—then contact your endocrinologist for help in adjusting your insulin levels.

Morning sickness. The nausea and vomiting associated with morning sickness can make it very difficult to eat right and maintain stable blood sugars. For most women, morning sickness occurs in the first trimester and tapers off during the second trimester, meaning it isn't much of a problem for women with gestational diabetes. However, women with type 1 diabetes may find it very challenging to have steady blood sugar levels during this time. Low blood sugar levels can make the problem worse, and many women find it helpful to nibble on crackers or dry toast when they feel nauseous. Again, be sure to test regularly—that's the only way you can be sure your blood sugar levels are neither high nor low. It may also be easier to eat smaller, more frequent meals.

Watch your weight. Pregnant women—both those with diabetes and those without—typically gain about 30 pounds during the course of pregnancy. Some diabetic women make such an effort to control their diabetes that they inadvertently lose weight, which can put the pregnancy at risk. Test your urine for ketones every morning to make sure you are not losing weight by burning fat. As noted earlier, this can possibly jeopardize your pregnancy. Contact your doctor immediately if you detect ketones in your urine.

Limit breakfast carbs. Many women struggle to maintain blood sugar balance after breakfast, often because it takes time for the first dose of insulin in the morning to take effect. Limit carbohydrates at breakfast. Consider having a small breakfast and a mid-morning snack to spread the carbohydrates out over the morning.

Eat before bed. Pregnant diabetic women should have a snack before bed because the baby will continue to need glucose during the overnight hours. If you don't eat, you risk allowing your blood sugar to go too low. You should combine some protein with the carbohydrate to slow the absorption and avoid a spike in blood sugar. Common bedtime snacks include graham crackers and milk, ice cream, and apple slices with peanut butter. Talk to your doctor or a dietician about your specific meal plan.

Exercise—with caution. Moderate exercise is good during pregnancy, and it can help you maintain stable blood sugar levels, in addition to keeping you strong, controlling weight gain, easing constipation, and improving your overall outlook. Women at risk for premature labor should not exercise at all, but most women can enjoy moderate exercise, especially if they were accustomed to regular workouts before conception. Talk to your obstetrician about designing a pregnancy exercise plan. Always test your blood sugar before exercise and keep a source of fast-acting carbohydrates with you at all times to avoid low blood sugars. Do not exercise if your blood sugar is over 200, since this can make your blood sugar rise even higher.

Don't panic if you go low. If you experience hypoglycemia—a low blood sugar insulin reaction—don't worry about what it could do to your baby. The placenta provides glucose to the baby even if the mother's blood sugar is too low. Obviously, you need to treat the situation immediately, but don't make matters worse by fretting about any possible damage to the developing fetus.

Choosing an obstetrician. If possible, choose an obstetrician with experience working with diabetic women. You will need to continue to see your endocrinologist as well, but the obstetrician will have expertise in monitoring the baby's health. Diabetic mothers are classified as having high-risk pregnancies, so you should not minimize the importance of working with the best medical team you can find.

Timing of delivery. Obstetricians used to try to deliver babies early if the mother had diabetes, but now most prefer to allow the pregnancy to go full term (as long as the mother has had reasonably good blood sugar control so the baby isn't too large). Doctors now have the ability to test to determine if the baby is mature for delivery. Although every attempt should be made to allow the pregnancy to go full term, you should be aware that the rate of cesarean section is three to five times higher among women with diabetes compared to women who do not have the disease.

Treating Diabetes During Pregnancy

During pregnancy, you can control diabetes with diet, exercise, and insulin—but no oral medications. The oral hypoglycemic agents used to treat type 2 diabetics cannot be used by pregnant women because of their possible impact on the developing fetus. Women with type 2 diabetes and gestational diabetes may need to use insulin to control their blood sugar during pregnancy, just as women with type 1 diabetes do.

Don't worry if your doctor recommends the use of insulin to control your blood sugar. Remember, you're doing this to protect the health of your unborn child. Is there any better motivator than that? If you didn't need insulin before your pregnancy, you probably won't need it afterward.

Some women require two injections while others need three or four injections a day to cover meals and the background insulin during the 24-hour period. (For information on insulin, see Chapter 7.) Your doctor will be able to assess your insulin demands and recommend a treatment plan based on the needs of you and your baby. Taking four injections doesn't mean your situation is any "worse" than someone taking two injections a day. Your doctor will be able to adjust your routine based on how your body is handling the insulin demands throughout the day.

Women with type 1 diabetes often find an insulin pump particularly beneficial during pregnancy because they can administer small amounts of insulin many times during the day to provide tight control. (For more information on pump therapy, see Chapter 8.)

Whether you're using injections or a pump, you need to be aware of how to administer insulin to correct for unexpected high blood sugars. Your doctor will be able to provide clear instructions on exactly how much insulin to administer to bring down your blood sugar. For example, you may be told to take 1 unit of insulin for every 50 mg/dL you are above 100.

Your insulin demands will change throughout your pregnancy, largely due to changes in hormone levels. At about 8 to 12 weeks of pregnancy, many women with type 1 diabetes require less insulin. From 12 weeks to delivery, insulin demands steadily increase. In other words, you will need to constantly adjust your insulin treatment to maintain stable blood sugar levels. Then brace yourself: Your insulin demands will drop back to your prepregnancy level shortly after the baby is born.

It is essential to maintain good blood sugar control during labor and delivery. During labor, most women need very little insulin because of the hard work they are doing. If your blood sugar is too high, the baby will produce too much insulin and go low after delivery. If your blood sugar is too low, then your baby may produce ketones during delivery. Many doctors will provide intravenous insulin and glucose to try to maintain balance.

Breastfeeding is good for mother and baby. If you have type 1 diabetes, you will need to eat more—and possibly take less insulin—because the baby will take glucose from you by nursing. Check your blood sugar before breastfeeding and have a snack, such as a glass of milk, a piece of fruit, or a few crackers. If you feel hypoglycemic, stop breastfeeding and test again. You may need a second snack, depending on your blood sugar numbers and how much milk you are producing. You should work with your doctor and, once again, test your blood sugar frequently to determine what your physical needs are.

Whether you have gestational or pregestational diabetes, making it through a pregnancy with diabetes can be challenging, although the ultimate reward of a healthy baby will be well worth the effort. Frequent blood sugar testing is absolutely essential so that you can keep your sugar levels as stable as possible. By working with your doctor and carefully managing your diabetes, you can go a long way toward providing for your baby, even before he or she is born.

In addition to making it through pregnancy safely, many pregnant women who have diabetes worry about the long-term consequences of living with diabetes. The following section outlines the complications that can occur if you have poor blood sugar control. Fortunately, if you practice good self-care and careful diabetes management, most complications can be avoided.

PART III
COMPLICATIONS

CHAPTER 14
COMMON COMPLICATIONS: An Overview

David knew he should go to the doctor for annual physicals, but he allowed years—almost twenty years—to go by between the time he saw a doctor for a life insurance physical and when he went back because he felt weak and he was seeing spots in front of his eyes whenever he bent over. He knew that he had allowed himself to get out of shape, but he was genuinely surprised to learn that he had extremely high blood pressure, early stage neuropathy (numbness in his feet)—and type 2 diabetes. "I started to have complications before I even knew I had diabetes," David said.

Kate, on the other hand, had lived with type 1 diabetes since she was in elementary school. She had a difficult time during her teens and early twenties, and she did not care for herself or her diabetes very well. By the time she was 22, she had serious vision problems. "Everyone told me it was going to happen, but I thought all the problems wouldn't happen until I was old," said Kate, now in her late twenties. "I guess I was in denial, because I really didn't think it would happen to me."

As both David and Kate now know, anyone with diabetes who does not maintain healthy blood sugar levels can be at risk of developing complications. These complications can involve your blood vessels, brain, eyes, heart, kidneys, legs and feet, and nerves.

As a general rule, your risk of complications increases when your blood sugar levels go above 200. The higher the level and the longer you remain in the danger zone, the greater your risk of developing problems. The best way to avoid complications is to keep your weight down and your blood sugar in the normal range. The closer your blood sugar levels are to normal, the more likely you can prevent or delay any complications.

A Look at the Research

The Diabetes Control and Complications Trial was a 10-year study sponsored by the National Institutes of Health. When it ended in 1993, it showed that people with type 1 diabetes who kept their blood sugar levels in the same range as those of people without diabetes had dramatically fewer complications than those with high blood sugar levels.

The researchers looked at 1,441 people with type 1 diabetes. Some of the study participants used standard therapy (one or two injections a day), and others followed an intensive therapy (three or more times a day or an insulin pump). In general, those on the more intensive therapy had blood sugar levels closer to normal and fewer complications—76 percent fewer cases of eye disease, 60 percent fewer cases of nerve damage, and 35 to 56 percent fewer cases of kidney damage than the group that used standard therapy.

The United Kingdom Prospective Diabetes Study followed 5,102 people with type 2 diabetes for an average of 10 years. These participants were divided into conventional and intensive groups, and people in both groups used insulin and oral medications in various combinations. The people in the intensive group, which maintained tighter control of their blood sugar, reduced their risk of heart attack, eye disease, kidney disease, and nerve disease. In addition, those study participants who also maintained good control of their blood pressure had a reduced risk of stroke, heart failure, vision loss, and other diabetic complications. The evidence is clear: It pays to control your blood sugar levels.

What High Blood Sugar Does to Your Body

In one of the waiting rooms at my daughter's endocrinologist's office, I saw a visual aid that compared the viscosity, or thickness, of fluids representing various blood sugar levels. The fluid representing normal blood sugar flowed quickly and smoothly, like sugar water. The fluid representing high blood sugar was thick and slow moving, like corn syrup. By visualizing the physical change in the blood that accompanied the elevation in blood sugar, I could easily imagine how the thick, sticky, high-sugar blood could clog up the blood vessels and make a mess of the circulatory system.

High blood sugar can cause both immediate and long-term problems:

- Immediate complications are the body's warning signs that the blood sugar is too high. These include thirst, frequent urination, blurred vision, and fatigue, and they usually disappear as soon as the blood sugar returns to normal. In extreme situations, they can result in coma or ketoacidosis (discussed in detail in the next chapter).

• Long-term complications reflect damage to the body caused by chronic high blood sugars, and often these problems cannot be reversed. It often takes years or decades for high blood sugar to cause long-term complications.

In the past, many people with diabetes experienced long-term complications. Fortunately, doctors now know much more about how to treat diabetes, and we have much better treatments and methods of monitoring blood sugar levels than people did a generation ago. Many of the people who experienced heartbreaking complications lived for decades with excessively high blood sugar levels.

With the screening tools and products available today, you can learn to manage your diabetes and minimize your risk of complications. Maintaining healthy blood sugar levels does matter. In addition, by working with your doctor, you can also identify and treat various problems as soon as they appear. For example, the damage caused by diabetic eye disease can often be minimized if the problem is detected and treated in its earliest stages.

Serious complications of diabetes are not inevitable. The information provided in this section will help you learn how to identify and treat potential problems if and when they first appear. The following chapter covers the short-term complications of excessively high blood sugar, including ketoacidosis and diabetic coma.

CHAPTER 15
DIABETIC CRISIS: Ketoacidosis and Coma

Just after the first bell rang, Kelly, a high school junior, realized that she hadn't changed the infusion set on her insulin pump. She knew she didn't have enough insulin to last through the entire afternoon, but she had a lot of important classes that day and she didn't want to take time away from school to deal with it.

She didn't think going a couple of hours without insulin would really matter. She was wrong. She noticed that she was thirsty and she needed to use the bathroom more than usual. By lunchtime, her blood sugar was over 400. She had to call her mother, who came to school and brought the supplies necessary to replenish the insulin in Kelly's pump. If Kelly had let her blood sugar stay high, she could have ended up in the hospital.

Whenever your blood sugar is high for several hours, you are at risk of developing diabetic ketoacidosis (DKA) or hyperosmolar coma, two potentially life-threatening diabetic complications.

Ketoacidosis occurs when the body produces too many ketones. Ketones are nothing more than the chemical by-product of fat breakdown, which occurs all the time in the body. Problems arise, however, when the body burns more fat than normal, such as when you don't eat for 12 hours or more—or, in the case of diabetics, when the blood sugar is too high and the body burns fat for energy because it doesn't have enough insulin to use the sugar in the blood.

Ketones are themselves acidic, and an excessively high level of ketones can change the pH balance of the body, leaving it too acidic. This highly acidic state is referred to as ketoacidosis. Left untreated, the condition will cause organ damage and ultimately death.

Taking insulin is the key to avoiding high blood sugar and ketoacidosis. Insulin allows the body to use the sugar in the bloodstream so that the body does not turn to stored fat as its only source of energy.

People who do not have diabetes can also have ketones in their urine and blood. In a non-diabetic person, the body uses carbohydrates from food for energy, then stores away any extra carbohydrates as fat for use in the future. In other words, it uses the carbs in the food first, and the stored fat second. When the fat is burned, some ketones will be produced, and a small amount may spill into the urine. While ketones are present, the level is not significant enough to damage the body. This is not ketoacidosis. (Some diet plans encourage you to test your urine for ketones as a sign that you are burning fat.)

Warning Signs of Ketoacidosis

It is important to be aware of the symptoms, since ketoacidosis can occur within several hours. In addition to the classic symptoms of high blood sugar—thirst, frequent urination, and fatigue—ketoacidosis can cause shortness of breath, a condition sometimes referred to as "air hunger." Heavy deep breathing, similar to breathing after exercise, is another way the body tries to rid itself of excess acid. The breath may smell sweet or fruity. Ketones can also cause nausea and vomiting. Since the symptoms of ketoacidosis can mimic symptoms of flu or other illnesses, it is essential that you test your blood sugar regularly whenever you are sick.

In addition, your doctor can write a prescription for Ketostix, reagent strips for urinalysis, which allow you to test at home to determine if you are spilling ketones in your urine. When urine wets the sticks, the tip of the stick changes color, from tan to pink to dark burgundy, indicating whether the amount of ketones is negative, trace, small, moderate, or large. You and your doctor should have a plan for when you should seek medical attention. My daughter's endocrinologist recommends that we call her if her ketones are "small" and seek medical care if the level is "moderate" or higher.

Causes of Ketoacidosis

At the most basic level, ketoacidosis occurs when a person with diabetes does not have enough insulin. In some cases, a diabetic may not be injecting enough insulin, or the insulin may have gone bad. Problems arise when a diabetic does not have access to insulin or the supplies needed to administer it safely. If blood sugar levels go high enough and stay high for several hours, a person with diabetes will develop ketoacidosis.

Illness can trigger a temporary—although sometimes dramatic—rise in blood sugar levels. In some cases, blood sugar levels rise even before the first symptoms of colds or flu appear. Stomach upset can be particularly challenging, since it can be difficult to balance carbohydrate intake and insulin damages when you're vomiting and therefore not sure how much food has been consumed. Frequent blood sugar monitoring is essential during periods of illness. (For more information on sick days, see Chapter 25.) To prevent ketoacidosis, you must continue to take insulin when you are sick, even if you aren't able to eat full meals.

Treatment for Ketoacidosis

Ketoacidosis is a medical emergency; it should be treated by a doctor in a hospital. In many cases, intravenous fluids are required to balance the electrolytes, maintain proper hydration, and administer insulin to bring the blood sugar back down. With medical attention, ketoacidosis can be treated in most situations. Without appropriate treatment, the condition can be fatal. Do not hesitate to seek care at the hospital emergency room if you experience symptoms of ketoacidosis.

Hyperosmolar Coma

You may have heard the term "diabetic coma," a term that dates back to the years before the introduction of insulin as a treatment for diabetes. In the pre-insulin years, children and young adults with type 1 diabetes often slipped into a ketoacidosis-induced coma prior to death. Fortunately, we now have treatments that can be used to treat ketoacidosis before it becomes life-threatening. This type of diabetic coma is not the same as a hyperosmolar coma.

If your blood sugar goes high enough, your body can begin to shut down and go into a hyperosmolar coma (also known as hyperosmolar hyperglycemic nonketotic syndrome, or HHNS). This typically does not occur unless the blood sugar level is more than 600, and it can be as high as an astounding 2,000 mg/dL. Blood sugar levels can climb to these frightening heights because as the blood sugar rises, the body tries to pass the sugar to the urine, causing dehydration. Water drains from all over the body to dilute the urine, causing intense thirst and further dehydration.

Symptoms of hyperosmolar coma include blood sugar levels over 600, dry mouth, extreme thirst, dry skin (no sweat), high fever, sleepiness, loss of vision, hallucinations, and weakness on one side of the body.

Hyperosmolar coma is more common in people with type 2 diabetes than type 1, because people with type 1 typically develop ketoacidosis before the situation reaches the crisis point. Hyperosmolar coma is a medical emergency that demands immediate attention. Untreated, it can be fatal.

Hyperosmolar coma can be prevented by testing blood sugar regularly and treating high blood sugar before it becomes dangerous. Frequent testing is especially important if you are sick because fever and vomiting can exacerbate dehydration.

Ketoacidosis is a short-term medical crisis, but many other complications occur more gradually over a longer period of time. The following chapter discusses eye problems and blindness, which can occur if you have poorly controlled diabetes over a long period of time.

CHAPTER 16
EYE PROBLEMS AND BLINDNESS

One of the most feared complications of diabetes is blindness. This fear is not misplaced: Diabetes is the most common cause of new blindness in adults from age 20 to 74. After 20 years with diabetes, nearly all people with type 1 diabetes show signs of eye disease and more than half of all people with type 2 diabetes develop diabetes-related vision problems.

Now the good news: There is a great deal that you can do to prevent eye problems, and if you find and treat eye problems early, most diabetic retinopathy doesn't cause any loss of vision.

How Your Eyes Work

In a healthy eye, the retina picks up the image you're focusing on and sends it to the brain. The image passes through the cornea (the clear cover over the pupil) and the pupil (the black part of the eye), where it is focused by the lens. Vision problems can occur if the lens doesn't work right (meaning you need glasses or contact lenses), if the lens is cloudy (meaning you need cataract surgery), or if this part of the eye is under pressure (meaning you have glaucoma). None of these vision problems is caused by diabetes.

Diabetes can cause problems with the vitreous gel, a substance that helps to keep the eyeball spherical. When the vitreous gel is clear, the image can be focused on the macula, the central area of retina responsible for vision. (The sides of the retina are used for peripheral vision.) When blood invades the vitreous gel, the image cannot get through to the retina.

Vitreous bleeding doesn't happen all at once. It occurs after years of diabetic retinopathy. The problem usually first appears as background retinopathy, meaning micro-aneurysms, or small red spots, have started to form on the retina. The problem can also appear as larger smudges known as microhemorrhages or yellowish deposits known as exudates.

Don't panic if your eye doctor reports that you have signs of background retinopathy. This problem usually occurs in 50 percent of people after having diabetes for 7 years and about 90 percent after 15 years. Background retinopathy is not dangerous and will not in itself cause impaired vision in most cases.

Vision problems become a greater threat if the condition progresses to proliferative retinopathy, the next stage in which additional blood vessels form in the eye. If these delicate vessels break, blood can leak into the vitreous gel, causing impaired vision or blindness within hours. Over a period of months, the blood will usually drain and vision will be restored. However, repeated bleeds can cause scarring and permanent damage to the retina.

Warning Signs of Diabetic Eye Disease

The early stages of diabetic eye disease do not have symptoms, making it absolutely essential that you have regular eye exams so that your doctor can diagnose and treat eye disease at the earliest stages. Early treatment can help to reduce the changes of permanent vision problems later on.

Most endocrinologists recommend annual eye exams for people who have had type 1 diabetes for more than five years and for everyone with type 2 diabetes since the condition may have been present for years prior to diagnosis. Look for an ophthalmologist with experience treating diabetics, since he or she will know how to look for the signs of diabetic retinopathy.

To test for background retinopathy, your doctor will need to dilate your pupils and conduct an eye test. (A comprehensive assessment cannot be done without dilating the eyes.) At the early stages, a visual exam is usually all that is necessary. Once there is evidence that vessels have formed in the eye, the ophthalmologist may use fluorescent angiography to look for leaking vessels. During the procedure, the doctor injects yellow dye into a vein and takes a series of retinal pictures to assess the condition of the vessels. The dye turns the urine yellow and can make some people nauseous, but it causes no long-term side effects.

Causes of Diabetic Eye Disease

Good blood sugar control is at the heart of preventing diabetic eye disease. Balanced blood sugar levels help stop diabetic retinopathy from occurring in the first place, and it helps slow the progression of the disease once it has been identified. In other words, it's never too late to get serious about watching your blood sugar. Your good vision depends on good blood sugar control.

Treatment for Diabetic Eye Disease

Diabetic eye disease can be treated if caught early.

- Photocoagulation involves using a laser beam to coagulate or block the vessels that may cause vitreous bleeding if left untreated. During the procedure, a doctor dilates the pupil, numbs the eye, and burns tiny spots on the retina using a laser. Because the eye is numbed, the procedure is not particularly painful, although the eye may feel achy and sore after the anesthetic wears off. Several studies have found that laser photocoagulation reduces vision loss by 90 percent or more.

- Vitrectomy involves surgically removing the vitreous gel and replacing it with a synthetic gel. The procedure is performed only when vision has been impaired by problems from recurring episodes of bleeding. The success of the surgery depends on the existing damage to the eyes and on whether the bleeding occurs again in the replacement gel.

In addition to having regular eye exams, you should contact your doctor if your vision becomes blurry, you have trouble reading, you see double, one or both eyes hurt, you feel pressure in your eyes, you see spots or floaters, or you lose your peripheral vision. These can be

signs of eye disease, and you should have your ophthalmologist examine your eyes.

Another common long-term complication of diabetes
is cardiovascular disease. The following chapter discusses
the link between diabetes and heart and circulatory disease.

CHAPTER 17
CARDIOVASCULAR DISEASE

Poor blood sugar control puts you at risk of developing cardiovascular disease. People with diabetes are two to four times more likely to get heart disease and five times more likely to have a stroke compared to people who do not have diabetes. In fact, cardiovascular disease causes more than half of the deaths of older people with diabetes.

Understanding Cardiovascular Disease

Arteriosclerosis, also known as hardening of the arteries, is characterized by the formation of fatty plaque deposits on the walls of the arteries. As the plaque builds up, the opening narrows, restricting blood flow. This increases blood pressure and will ultimately result in a blockage.

Arteriosclerosis can affect the blood supply to the heart (heart disease), the legs (peripheral vascular disease), and the brain (cerebrovascular disease). Heart disease is the most common problem caused by hardening of the arteries. The coronary arteries supply blood to the heart muscle. When these arteries are blocked, some of the heart tissue dies. Arteriosclerosis blocks the coronary arteries.

If the coronary artery is partly blocked, the heart may get enough blood while at rest, but not enough during periods of exertion or stress. This condition is known as angina pectoris, and it is characterized by pain during exercise and times of physical or emotional stress. The pain eases when the heart rate slows. Consult a doctor if you experience symptoms of angina.

Peripheral vascular disease affects the arteries in the legs and feet. When these arteries are partly blocked, the calf and thigh muscles can hurt during exercise because they aren't getting enough oxygen. This condition, known as claudication, is similar to angina, only it involves the legs rather than the heart. If the artery is completely blocked, the leg tissue can die, causing gangrene and the loss of the limb. This doesn't happen often because the body usually develops secondary arteries to bypass the blockage.

Cerebrovascular disease affects the arteries in the brain. Partial blockages cause transient ischemic attacks (TIAs), which can cause temporary neurological problems, such as a numb arm or problems with speech. These problems usually disappear after a few minutes, but they can recur. Complete blockage of an artery in the brain causes a stroke, or the death of a part of the brain when it has been deprived of oxygen.

While these conditions can be frightening, some degree of arteriosclerosis happens to almost everyone. There are approaches that can reduce the risk of serious problems, and drugs and surgical procedures that can help to clear the arteries if the blockages become severe.

Warning Signs of Cardiovascular Disease

Chest pain in the form of angina or leg pain indicating peripheral vascular disease is the typical first sign of circulatory diseases. That said, many people don't have any warning before they experience their first heart attack.

You should always be vigilant about responding to the signs of a heart attack. Most heart attack deaths occur in the first two hours, yet studies have found that many people wait four to six hours to get to an emergency room. Do not ignore the warning signs of a heart attack, including:

- Chest pain: an uncomfortable pressure, fullness, squeezing, or crushing feeling in the center of the chest that lasts two minutes or longer

- Severe pain that radiates to the shoulders, neck, arms, jaw, or top of the stomach

- Shortness of breath

- Paleness

- Sweating

- Rapid or irregular pulse

- Dizziness, fainting, or loss of consciousness

Not all warning signs occur when you have a heart attack. Some people don't experience warning signs at all. If you think you may have heart problems, consult a doctor. If you think you may be having a heart attack, go to the emergency room immediately.

If you experience pain in your legs when exercising, contact your doctor so that you can be screened for peripheral vascular disease. Similarly, if you experience recurring neurological symptoms, such as numbness in one arm or short-term strokelike symptoms, contact your doctor immediately, even if the episodes only last for a minute or two. The earlier you seek medical care, the more likely you will be to avoid a more serious problem later.

Causes of Cardiovascular Disease

There are several known factors that put you at greater risk of developing cardiovascular disease, including poor control of diabetes, high cholesterol, high blood pressure, smoking, and family history of heart disease. In addition, aging and menopause also increase your risk. Some factors you can control; others you can't, but the more risk factors you have, the greater your likelihood of developing cardiovascular problems.

Treatment for Cardiovascular Disease

If you have signs of cardiovascular disease, you should be under the care of a specialist. Talk to your endocrinologist about getting a referral. In addition to following your doctor's advice, you should follow the basics of good cardiovascular self-care.

Maintain good blood sugar control. High blood sugar increases your risk of arteriosclerosis.

Watch your cholesterol. Have your cholesterol checked at your annual physical exam. Strive to keep your LDL cholesterol and triglycerides low and your HDL cholesterol high. (LDL cholesterol causes arteriosclerosis, while HDL cholesterol helps prevent it.) Aim for LDL cholesterol under 100 mg/dL and HDL over 50 mg/dL. Talk to your doctor about how to use diet and medication to meet your cholesterol goals.

Keep your blood pressure at a healthy level. If your blood pressure is over 140/80, take steps to bring it down. Shedding extra pounds if you're overweight, exercising regularly, and avoiding salt in the diet can be helpful. Your doctor may also prescribe medication to lower your blood pressure. A class of drugs known as ACE inhibitors are often used to reduce blood pressure in people who have diabetes, but the drugs also help slow the progression of kidney disease.

If you smoke, quit. The nicotine in cigarette smoke constricts the blood vessels, interfering with the flow of oxygen and nutrients to the cells. Smoking is one of the toughest addictions to shake, but about half of all Americans alive today who have smoked have managed to quit. Support programs can make a difference. Low-cost or free programs are offered by many hospitals, as well as the American Lung Association and the American Cancer Society. You can do it.

If you have a family history of heart disease, make a special effort to reduce other risk factors. Of course, you want to take every step possible to reduce all your risk factors, but you should be especially careful if your father or brother developed hardening of the arteries before age 55 or your mother or sister before age 65.

Another chronic complication of diabetes is nerve damage or neuropathy, which can cause serious problems for people with diabetes. Diabetic neuropathy and its warning signs are discussed in the following chapter.

CHAPTER 18
DIABETIC NEUROPATHY

Mara suspected she had type 2 diabetes several years before she went to her doctor for help. At first her feet felt tingly, especially at night. Over the years, the problem became more pronounced and eventually she lost most of the sensation in her toes. Mara knew that diabetes could cause foot problems, but she avoided her doctor because she didn't want the condition to be diagnosed. She was more than 100 pounds overweight and an admitted junk-food addict, and Mara didn't want to make the necessary lifestyle changes to improve her health.

When the problem reached the point that she could no longer ignore the numbness in her feet, Mara made an appointment with her doctor. She felt ashamed and frightened, but her endocrinologist was able to teach her how to manage her diabetes and to practice good foot care. While she remains anxious about the prospect of losing a toe or a part of a toe, she now realizes that the only way to avoid serious complications is to work to control her blood sugar levels.

Diabetic neuropathy, or nerve damage, is a long-term

complication of diabetes. In some cases, people like Mara already have some nerve damage at the time they are diagnosed with type 2 diabetes, but these people have typically lived with high blood sugar for a number of years before diagnosis. About 60 to 70 percent of people with diabetes have mild to severe forms of neuropathy.

Diabetic neuropathy involves damage to the nervous system. Each nerve is an individual line or thread that connects to the spine and carries nerve impulses up to the brain. Billions of these threads, known as axons, run throughout the body. The longest connect the spine and the toes.

There are two basic types of nerves—sensory nerves, which provide information about pain, temperature, and body position, and motor nerves, which provide information about muscle movement. If the sensory nerves are damaged, a person won't feel pain and can experience injury without knowing it. If the motor nerves are damaged, the body can experience problems with autonomic muscle systems, including sexual dysfunction and digestive problems, among others.

Diabetic neuropathy usually involves the sensory nerves. When the nerves are irritated, the sensory messages don't carry messages reliably, causing pain, sensitivity, or numbness. Nerves recover from injury very slowly, if at all, so it is much better to avoid nerve damage than to expect the body to repair itself after the fact.

Warning Signs of Diabetic Neuropathy
Diabetic neuropathy usually develops 10 years or more after diagnosis. Diabetics who maintain good blood sugar

control may go decades—or their entire lives—without developing neuropathy, so the problem should not be considered an inevitable complication of diabetes. There are three main types of neuropathy: peripheral, autonomic, and single-nerve.

Peripheral neuropathy involves the sensory nerves in the feet and hands. It typically starts as tingling or numbness in the toes. Over a period of years, those feelings travel up to the ankle and leg. The condition almost always occurs on both feet rather than on one side or the other.

Symptoms can be mild or severe. Some people aren't aware of symptoms until a doctor tests their reflexes. Other people report that their feet are either too sensitive (even the feeling of sheets on the bed can be painful) or not sensitive enough (they can't feel anything at all). Usually, the overly sensitive stage passes as feelings of numbness spread.

Numbness can be particularly dangerous since the feet can be injured without the person knowing. Many people report that stray objects, such as tacks or other sharp items, can be left in shoes, and the person with neuropathy doesn't realize it until the end of the day, after the damage has been done. A new pair of shoes, a long walk, or stubbing a toe can cause ulcers and foot damage, which can, in extreme cases or if left untreated, lead to amputation. (For more information on foot problems and amputations, see Chapter 19.)

Autonomic neuropathy affects the nerves of the autonomic nervous system, which are responsible for involuntary muscle movement. This can cause a number of problems, such as:

- Impotence in men and a lack of sexual responsiveness in women

- Bowel problems, typically alternating periods of constipation and diarrhea

- Urinary retention, which can cause kidney damage if urine backs up to the kidneys

- Gastroparesis, or damage to the nerves in the stomach, which can cause the stomach to empty erratically, making good blood sugar control very difficult

- Dizziness when standing up (orthostasis)

- Sweating disorders, in which some parts of the bodies do not sweat and others sweat too much

Autonomic neuropathy occurs in 20 to 40 percent of people with long-standing diabetes.

Single-nerve neuropathy or mononeuropathy involves damage to a single nerve when the blood supply is cut off, almost as if the nerve experiences a small stroke. With single-nerve neuropathy, symptoms appear suddenly and affect only the part of the body involving the single nerve so the symptoms are not symmetrical. Most single-nerve neuropathies involve sensory nerves, but in some cases they can involve nerves that cause an eyelid to droop, for example. In most cases, single-nerve neuropathies resolve themselves and symptoms disappear in a matter of weeks or months.

Bell's palsy is a type of single-nerve neuropathy that causes one side of the face to droop. It is common in people with diabetes, although it can happen in non-diabetics as well.

In rare cases, several nerves can develop neuropathies at the same time. This condition, known as multiple single-nerve involvement, mononeuritis multiplex or mononeuropathy multiplex, can cause weakness in the hips and thighs to the point that a person cannot stand. Fortunately, this condition also improves, although it may take more than a year.

Causes of Diabetic Neuropathy

Most cases of diabetic neuropathy involve gradual damage to the nerves caused by chronic high blood sugar. The cells first affected tend to be those farthest from the spine—the toes. These nerve cells become damaged by swelling caused by build-up of sugar or proteins on the cells.

Single-nerve neuropathies are caused by loss of blood supply to a portion of the nerve. In these cases, the nerve itself is damaged or destroyed by the lack of nutrients to the tissue.

Treatment for Diabetic Neuropathy

Peripheral and autonomic neuropathies are effectively irreversible. This is because the nerve cells grow back very slowly, if at all.

That said, medications can be used to reduce the various symptoms caused by the neuropathies. For example, the antidepressant drugs mitriptyline and desipramine, as well as traditional pain medications, can be used to treat foot pain. Other drugs can be used to address problems with impotence and digestion, and other symptoms of neuropathy. The success of these treatments depends on the extent of the nerve damage.

Of course, it would be better to prevent the problems than to treat the symptoms after they occur. Current research is being done to assess the safety and efficacy of aldose reductase inhibiting drugs to block the accumulation of sugar on the cells, preventing or minimizing the risk of neuropathy. This treatment is under investigation, but it does not replace the need for good blood sugar control.

Many diabetics have heard frightening stories of people who have had toes or feet amputated as a last-resort treatment for complications associated with neuropathy. The following chapter examines advanced foot problems and amputations. While the topic can be difficult to consider, please remember that in most cases this situation can be avoided with good management of your diabetes.

CHAPTER 19
FOOT PROBLEMS AND AMPUTATION

Foot problems are one of the more common serious complications for people with diabetes. In most cases, amputations are not inevitable; as many as 70 percent of diabetes-related amputations can be prevented.

Warning Signs of Foot Problems

The classic early symptoms of foot problems are tingling or pain in the toes and feet, as well as strange sensations, such as the feeling of water running over the feet. As the nerve damage progresses, the toes or feet may become numb, which is much more dangerous because you may not be aware that your feet are being injured until the damage is done. You might step on a thumbtack and not realize it, or burn yourself by stepping into excessively hot bathwater without realizing the water temperature.

Causes of Foot Problems

Peripheral neuropathy (discussed in the previous chapter) and poor circulation are the main causes of diabetic foot problems. Poor circulation—peripheral vascular disease—also contributes to foot problems. When circulation is poor due to narrowing of the arteries caused by arteriosclerosis and smoking, then the tissues receive less blood, meaning they receive less oxygen, nutrients, and infection-fighting cells. The tissues aren't nourished and they are more likely to become infected and to have trouble healing.

In some cases, the shape of the foot can contribute to nerve problems, especially if an orthopedic problem causes the weight to be distributed unevenly. A podiatrist can analyze your feet for places to watch for problems, including spots with calluses or bunions. Be sure to wear comfortable shoes. Wearing tight shoes can cause pressure points that are vulnerable to irritation and infection.

The combination of numbness and poor healing puts the feet at a much greater risk of encountering injury and infection, and it makes it much harder for the feet to recover. Regular foot care is essential for diabetics with neuropathy and circulatory problems.

Losing sensation in the feet happens gradually, and only a doctor can assess the amount of nerve damage. Circulation can be measured in a number of ways. One simple way is to feel both feet. If the blood flow is limited in one foot, it may be cooler than the other because an artery is partially blocked. (Don't worry if you have two cold feet; that isn't a reliable sign.) Doctors have more sophisticated tests to measure the pulses in the feet, including Doppler tests (to listen to the blood flow) and angiograms (to see the blood flow by putting dye into the bloodstream and taking a series of X rays).

Treatment for Foot Problems

Foot problems should be treated at the earliest sign of redness or a break in the skin. Call your doctor immediately and begin treatment while the problem is still minor and easier to control.

If you have a break in the skin or an ulcer on your foot, your doctor may prescribe antibiotics. Minor infections can be treated with oral antibiotics, but more severe infections may require intravenous antibiotics at the hospital. As is true with any antibiotic treatment, you must complete the entire course of treatment, even if you look and feel better before taking all of the medication.

You may be told to stay off your feet and keep the infected area elevated. Do it. This helps the tissue heal faster. Yes, it's hard to sit still when you have a million things to do, but rest will help you get back on your feet faster than rushing the healing process and developing complications later on.

Your doctor will need to handle the debridement, or the removal of the dead tissue around the infected area. This skin must be removed to control the spread of the bacteria. In simple cases, it can be done in the doctor's office; in deep wounds, it may require surgery under anesthesia.

While the foot is healing, doctors often recommend protecting it with casts or special shoes. Some doctors will put a cast over an ulcer or wound to protect the area while new tissue grows. Orthotics or specially designed shoes may be recommended to spread the weight more evenly across the foot. Orthotics can be expensive, but they can be a medical necessity for many diabetics with foot problems.

In some cases, surgery may be required to spare the foot. When circulation is limited, your doctor may need to perform vascular surgery to improve blood flow. If you have bony feet or spots that frequently rub against your shoe, your doctor may recommend orthopedic surgery to change the structure of your foot.

Hyperbaric oxygen may be recommended to treat non-healing wounds on the feet. The treatment involves spending about 90 minutes in a chamber with high oxygen levels under high air pressure.

Amputations

As a last resort, amputations are sometimes necessary. Amputations are one of the most feared complications of diabetes, but in most cases the removal of bone can be avoided with good blood sugar control and vigilant foot care.

Most foot amputations follow some kind of break in the skin on the foot, which becomes infected. The initial causes can be injuries, pressure points, blisters, or burns. It can be something as innocent as a long walk on a hot beach, or as obviously damaging as an errant metal clip left in the bottom of a shoe. Tight shoes can cause red spots or blisters that later turn into ulcers that won't heal or become infected.

Left untreated, infections can move into the bone, a condition known as osteomyelitis. The condition can be tricky to diagnose since it may not show up on an X ray. It can be very hard to treat; infection in the bone doesn't respond well to antibiotics. In some cases, the bone must be removed to prevent the infection from further spreading.

Amputation may involve only a toe or a part of a toe, an entire foot, or, rarely, the foot and lower leg. It is better to lose a toe than wait too long and have an infection spread to the entire foot. Amputation is usually considered when an infection won't heal and when gangrene has set in, meaning the tissue is already dead. Gangrenous tissue can't be revived, and it leaves the body subject to more infection, so it must be removed.

An Ounce of Prevention
It is much easier to prevent diabetic foot problems than it is to treat them.

- Exercise to improve your circulation. When you exercise, your body actually develops new blood vessels to bypass blockages in the arteries and meet the body's demand for oxygen.

- If you smoke, quit. Talk to your doctor if you need help with smoking cessation.

- Wash and dry your feet carefully. (Bacteria and fungi like moist, warm places.)

- Examine your feet carefully at least once a day. You can't rely on foot pain to tell you when something's wrong, so a visual inspection is essential.

- Trim your toenails straight across and round the corners slightly with a file. It's easiest to tend to your toenails after bathing, when the nails are softer.

- Never, never cut your calluses or corns. If you have a problem, consult a podiatrist for help.

- Wear shoes at all times—and be sure they fit. Consult a podiatrist for specific advice on finding shoes that fit.

- Wear new shoes for only a couple of hours at a time to avoid blisters.

- Shake out your shoes before putting them on to make sure nothing is inside them.

- Wear clean socks without holes that fit well and don't bind.

- Consult a doctor at the first sign that something is wrong. Don't let little problems become big ones.

While less visible than foot problems, kidney disease can also be caused by poor diabetes control. The following chapter describes the warning signs of kidney disease and what you can do to control the problem.

CHAPTER 20
KIDNEY PROBLEMS

The majority of people with diabetes never develop kidney problems. Approximately one out of every three people with diabetes experience kidney trouble, and many of them develop problems only after living with diabetes for decades. Being vigilant about good blood sugar control can help you prevent kidney problems, and it can help to halt the progress of the disease among those people who do show signs of kidney involvement.

Warning Signs of Kidney Disease
The kidneys are the body's filters, which work day and night to rid your body of toxins. The toxins from the blood pass through the capillaries and enter the filters in the kidneys. When the tiny capillaries are clogged and don't filter the blood very well, they allow toxins to remain in your blood and some proteins from the blood to spill into the urine. For this reason, the first sign of kidney problems in diabetics is typically proteinuria, or the presence of protein in the urine. Protein leaks through the kidneys because the filters aren't working right.

Urine tests can be done with a reagent stick dipped in

the urine. If there's protein in the urine, the stick will change colors. A more sensitive test measures tiny amounts of the protein albumin in the urine. This can be done on a random sample or in a timed test, during which you collect all your urine over a 24-hour period.

Kidney involvement is defined as significant amounts of protein in the urine or more than one sample. Your doctor should screen for protein in the urine at your annual exam. If protein is present in the urine, follow-up tests may be required.

Causes of Kidney Disease

Diabetic kidney disease is caused by damage to the small blood vessels. In some diabetics, the nephrons, or tiny filters inside the kidneys, thicken and clog up. The gumming up of the system typically happens in the first decade of having diabetes, but the symptoms often don't appear until years later.

The kidneys are designed to cleanse the blood by filtering out waste products. As the blood flows through the kidneys, it passes through millions of tiny filters. The waste products go into the urine, and the clean blood circulates throughout the body.

In addition, the kidneys regulate salt and water levels in the body. To maintain the appropriate balance, the kidneys excrete or retain water and salt as needed. The kidneys also help to regulate blood pressure. If you retain salt or fluid, your blood vessels become too full, like a bloated garden hose. This is hypertension, or high blood pressure. If the vessels are underfilled, it is hypotension, or low blood pressure. The kidneys help to keep the blood pressure just right.

Treatment for Kidney Disease

If you develop kidney disease, there are several issues you need to address to manage the problem, including controlling blood sugar and blood pressure.

You need to keep your blood sugar levels in balance to control kidney disease. High blood sugar levels—as measured by an A1c level over 8 percent—contribute to kidney damage. (For details on A1c levels, see Chapter 5.) The lower the average sugar level, the less likely you will develop kidney disease. Occasional bouts of high blood sugar probably won't cause problems. Focus on controlling blood sugar by keeping your average blood sugar levels as low as you can.

Hypertension can exacerbate kidney problems so you must keep your blood pressure in a healthy range. Strive to keep your blood pressure below 140/80. (The first number—the systolic number—is the pressure when the heart beats, the second number—the diastolic number—is the pressure when the heart is at rest.) If you feel dizzy when you stand up or can't go about your daily activities, your blood pressure may be too low.

In some cases, your doctor may prescribe ACE (angiotensin converting enzyme) inhibitors, drugs used to lower blood pressure and treat kidney disease. These drugs block a chemical reaction in the kidneys' control of blood pressure. Various drugs have different side effects and different durations, so your doctor may prescribe several before finding the right one. Researchers have found that people respond better to ACE inhibitors than other blood pressure medications. Some doctors prescribe ACE inhibitors to diabetic patients with proteinuria whether or not they have high blood pressure.

To minimize kidney problems, you should also watch what you eat. In addition to watching carbs, you will want to limit your salt intake if you have high blood pressure. If you develop proteinuria, limit protein to 10 or 12 percent of calories. Excessive protein can strain the kidneys.

Complications of Kidney Disease
Untreated, kidney disease can progress into serious health problems.

Kidney Failure
It is essential that you take steps to control proteinuria at the earliest stages to avoid kidney failure. In many cases of good control, signs of kidney failure won't show up for 10 or 15 years or longer. Approximately 43 percent of new cases of kidney failure are caused by diabetes.

At some point, kidney damage leads to end-stage renal disease or kidney failure. A lab test for creatine clearance assesses kidney function based on a 24-hour urine sample. A rate of about 100 milliliters per minute or more is normal; a rate of about 50 milliliters indicates kidney function about 50 percent of normal. Symptoms typically show up once creatine clearance drops to 20 or 30 milliliters per minute and dialysis or kidney transplant may be considered when levels drop to 15 milliliters or less.

Symptoms include ankle swelling (which can be caused by other conditions as well), anemia, fatigue, itching, nausea, and low urine production. This happens when the kidneys cannot clear the toxins from the blood adequately.

When the kidneys stop functioning, dialysis and transplantation are the available treatments. Dialysis—a machine that filters the blood of toxins—can be done at a dialysis center several times a week or with equipment at home.

Kidney transplants are sometimes combined with pancreas transplants. This is in essence a cure for diabetes, although it requires lifelong immunosuppressant medication, in addition to significant risks in the operation itself. Transplantation is not always successful, and there aren't nearly enough organs available to meet the demand. It is much safer to control diabetes than to rely on the possibility of receiving an organ transplant.

Diabetic kidney disease presents serious long-term problems, but it does not affect most people with diabetes. Those who do develop the condition can minimize the impact by controlling blood pressure and blood sugar levels.

Not every complication of diabetes is life-threatening. Poor control of diabetes can cause sexual dysfunction, including erectile dysfunction in men and diminished sexual desire, poor vaginal lubrication, and problems achieving orgasm in women. Sexual problems associated with diabetes are discussed in the following chapter.

CHAPTER 21
SEXUAL DYSFUNCTION

When Michael learned that he had type 2 diabetes at age 45, his first concern was the risk of developing impotence. "I was still a young man when I found out about my diabetes," he said. "I didn't want to 'retire' before my time."

Michael's concern about his sexual performance was not entirely unfounded. If you have poor blood sugar control, diabetes can interfere with your sexual function. Complications of diabetes can diminish libido, cause impotence, and reduce sexual responsiveness. Depression and other emotional challenges can create psychological barriers to sexual satisfaction, as well. When many people feel depressed, interest in sex is one of the first things to go, especially among diabetics.

Warning Signs of Sexual Dysfunction
Diabetes can cause impotence, vaginal infections, and fatigue, all of which can contribute to sexual problems.

For Women
• Poor vaginal lubrication can result from lower than normal estrogen levels, caused by chronic

high blood sugar over a period of months or years. Episodes of high blood sugar can also cause temporary bouts of vaginal dryness.

- Erratic menstrual periods can be caused by high blood sugar levels. It's best to rectify the problem by correcting blood sugar levels, but some doctors may prescribe birth control pills.

- Women may also experience neuropathy (described in Chapter 18), which can affect the genital area. Because the nerves become irritated or nonresponsive, women with neuropathy in the genital area may not be able to experience orgasm.

- Vaginal infections are common among women who have had high blood sugar for several days.

For Men
- Impotence is common in men with diabetes. The longer you have had diabetes and the less vigilant you have been about controlling your blood sugar, the greater the odds that you will develop impotence. Men with neuropathies also face greater risk.

Men and Impotence

Experiencing an erection takes a group effort: Your hormones, vascular system, and nervous system must be working together, and your head has to be in the game. Any number of physical or psychological issues can interfere with your ability to achieve and maintain an erection.

Psychological issues—particularly worry that you might be impotent—can contribute to sexual dysfunction. If you experience erectile problems inconsistently, if the problem occurs suddenly, if you have erections during the night and when you wake up, or if you do not have problems when you masturbate but do have problems when you're with a partner, you are more likely to have anxiety or psychological issues as part of the problem. If you never experience erections—even when you're asleep, bored, or masturbating—then it is more likely that your impotence is caused by a physical problem.

Your doctor can perform simple tests to determine whether or not you experience erections in your sleep. (Most men have an average of four erections during their sleep.) If there is no evidence of overnight erections, your doctor may perform additional tests to assess hormone levels and measure the health of your vascular and nervous systems.

Physical factors, particularly peripheral neuropathy, can also cause impotence. Peripheral neuropathy interferes with the body's ability to perceive the sensations associated with sexual contact. At first, impotence is usually partial, meaning it is difficult to maintain an erection, while over time the condition can become more complete, making it impossible to obtain an erection.

Causes of Sexual Dysfunction

On a short-term basis, high blood sugar levels make most people feel tired and lethargic, leaving them with little energy for sex. Thirst and frequent urination can also get in the way of romance. These acute problems tend to pass when blood sugar is brought back under control.

Chronic high blood sugars can lead to sexual dysfunction caused by vascular problems that limit the flow of blood into the genital area. Problems are more common among people with cardiovascular disease and poor circulation. Hardening of the arteries limits blood flow, making hardening of the penis increasingly difficult. Smoking can make vascular problems much worse; if you smoke, quit.

Some medications, such as blood pressure drugs (beta blockers and diuretics), antidepressants, and ulcer treatments, among others, can cause sexual problems as a side effect. Talk to your doctor about any changes you notice in your sexual responsiveness while on medication. In many cases, your doctor may be able to prescribe alternative medications that don't have the same side effects.

Treatment of Sexual Dysfunction

Fortunately, most temporary symptoms associated with sexual dysfunction will improve when the blood sugar level drops below 200. Once again, good blood sugar control is the key to good health.

Discuss the issue with your partner so that he or she will realize your limitations are physical and not a reflection of your feelings. Talk to your doctor, even if you have to raise the topic yourself. Studies have found that 85 percent of doctors asked their male patients about sex, but only 33 percent asked their female patients.

For women, vaginal dryness can be treated with topical ointments or estrogen replacement pills, patches, or creams. Vaginal lubricants can be used to lubricate and correct the pH balance in the vagina.

For men, talk to your doctors about various approaches

to treat impotence. Your doctor may prescribe a medication that is injected into the base of the penis to cause an erection that usually lasts about a half hour. Other approaches include using a vacuum device that encourages blood flow to the penis, or a surgical penile implant.

Impotence caused by poor blood flow often responds to yohimbine, a nutritional supplement that can be purchased at drug and health food stores. This approach should not be used by people with high blood pressure or cardiovascular disease without the recommendation of a doctor.

Whether you're a man or a woman, you should seek professional help if you are depressed. (Depression is discussed in detail in Chapter 24.) If you've explored some of the emotional challenges involving sexuality and you still have problems, consider speaking with a mental health professional with expertise in handling sexual concerns.

While sexual dysfunction and most of the other physical complications of diabetes occur inside your body, diabetes can also cause a number of skin problems, which are visible signs of the disease. These diabetic skin problems are discussed in the following chapter.

CHAPTER 22
SKIN PROBLEMS

People with diabetes can develop a number of different problems with their skin. Most of the skin problems are caused directly or indirectly by injecting insulin, and the rest are complications of chronic high blood sugar levels. If you experience symptoms, contact your endocrinologist or a dermatologist for help.

Acanthosis Nigricans

Acanthosis nigricans is a soft, velvety patch of dark skin that forms at the back of the neck and in the armpits of some people with type 2 diabetes. It is most common in people of African descent, although it can affect people of any race. The condition can also be a sign of insulin resistance. Consider the condition a warning sign of possible insulin problems. The skin condition does not cause any problems or require treatment on its own.

Alopecia (or Hair Loss)

Alopecia, or the loss of clumps of hair on the head, doesn't follow the classic patterns of balding. Instead of thinning and then creating gradual, even hair loss, alopecia causes clumps or clusters of hair to fall out. Some people with type 1 diabetes experience alopecia, especially when their blood sugars are not in good control and they are under significant stress. In most people with diabetes, the condition resolves itself when blood sugar control is reestablished.

Bruising

Injecting insulin can sometimes cause a small bruise at the injection site. This occurs when the needle pierces a blood vessel. In rare cases, some of the insulin can go directly into the bloodstream, rather than being absorbed through the subcutaneous fat. If this happens, you may experience a more rapid decline in blood sugar level.

Bruising can happen to anyone, but it is more common in people taking blood thinners, such as coumadin or daily aspirin. The bruise should resolve within a week to 10 days.

Dry Skin

While dry, overheated air is the primary cause of dry skin, the condition can be caused or made worse by high blood sugars. The high sugars can cause dehydration, which shows up in the skin, and in some cases autonomic nerve damage from chronic high sugars can cause a decrease in the activity of the sweat glands.

If dry skin is allowed to crack or break, it can put the body at increased risk of infection. This can be a serious problem if you have circulatory problems or neuropathy in your feet. Combat dry skin by drinking lots of water and using moisturizing lotions and soaps.

Fungal Infections

Fungus thrives in high-sugar environments. When you have poor blood sugar control, high sugars can encourage the growth of fungus under the toenails or between the toes. It can also appear as an itchy, red rash, especially in high moisture areas like the armpits, genital area, under the breasts, and in skin folds.

To eliminate fungal infections, control blood sugar and wash and dry the affected area carefully and thoroughly. Wear all-cotton underwear, which can be drier than synthetic fabrics. Athlete's foot (a fungal infection on the feet) can be treated with over-the-counter medications. Treat it at the earliest sign of infection, since entrenched infections can be more challenging to treat. If cracks form in the infected area, the infection can enter the body and spread. If a fungal infection doesn't respond to early treatment, contact a dermatologist for additional help.

Insulin Hypertrophy

Insulin hypertrophy is a patch of fatty tissue that forms in any area where you inject insulin frequently. Insulin actually encourages the formation of fatty tissue, but if you change injection (or infusion) sites regularly, there isn't enough insulin to make a noticeable difference.

Areas of insulin hypertrophy can be several inches across, or tiny patches. The tissue is soft (it's just fat) and painless, but you don't want to continue to use that spot as an injection site since it does not diffuse insulin as effectively as unaffected areas.

Lipoatrophy

One of the most frustrating parts of living with diabetes is that the disease can be maddeningly unpredictable. Just as hypertrophy causes the formation of fat under the skin, lipoatrophy causes the *loss* of fat under the skin—but both conditions are caused by injecting insulin into the same region too often. Lipoatrophy typically looks like a depressed area in the skin, and it may feel coarse or fibrous. As with patches of hypertrophy, the absorption of insulin may be unpredictable, so use another injection site.

Necrobiosis Lipoidica Diabeticorum

Necrobiosis lipoidica diabeticorum (NLD) is a skin condition that causes patches of purple skin. It occurs primarily in people with type 1 diabetes, usually within the first several years of diagnosis. The patches of affected skin are usually $\frac{1}{2}$ to 3 inches in diameter, most often on the shins, ankles, or feet. The patches appear over the course of several weeks, and they are not painful or irritating, although some people consider the affected areas unsightly. Over time, the patches often become depressed and brownish.

Pseudoscleroderma

Pseudoscleroderma causes thinning of the skin at the fingers and stiff finger joints. Unlike scleroderma, the condition doesn't seriously threaten health and will not become progressively worse. This condition is more common in people with diabetes than those with normal blood sugar levels.

Other musculoskeletal problems that occur more often in people with diabetes include tendon contractures in the palm of the hands, which can make it difficult to stretch out the fingers, and bursitis of the shoulder, elbows, knees, or hips.

Vitiligo

Vitiligo causes patches of skin to become stripped of all pigment. The condition is an autoimmune disease of the skin. The condition is more common among people with type 1 diabetes than others because people with one autoimmune condition seem to be susceptible to other autoimmune conditions as well.

If you develop vitiligo, contact a dermatologist to confirm the diagnosis. Be sure to wear sunscreen on the white patches, and avoid sun exposure to minimize the darkening of the surrounding skin.

Xanthelasma

Xanthelasma is a condition that causes the formation of small yellowish plaques in the corner of the eyes near the nose. The condition is hereditary, and it often accompanies diabetes. In some cases, xanthelasma occurs in people with high cholesterol.

Most of the skin problems associated with diabetes are temporary and not particularly serious. Some of these outward signs can provide important warnings of blood sugar imbalances, even before a person has been diagnosed with diabetes.

The following section, Living Well with Diabetes, can help you deal with the disease in your personal life, as well as at work and school. The next chapter, Finding the Right Health Care Providers, describes how to select and work with your health care team, including endocrinologists, dieticians, podiatrists, and other health-care providers.

PART IV

LIVING WELL WITH DIABETES

CHAPTER 23
FINDING THE RIGHT HEALTH-CARE PROVIDERS

If you have diabetes, you won't have one doctor but an entire health-care team. In addition to your primary care doctor, you will work with a doctor who handles your diabetes care, as well as other specialists who are focused on the specific challenges you face while managing your diabetes.

Consider yourself the captain of your health-care team. It's up to you to eat right, test your blood sugar often, and follow the doctors' orders, but you won't be alone in your efforts. You will probably have many of the following experts on your team.

• Primary care doctor: This is the doctor who coordinates your overall care and whose name is listed first on medical forms and on the slip of paper you should carry with you in your wallet. Most primary care doctors are internists or family practitioners. This person does not need to be an expert on diabetes but rather an expert on your overall health.

- Endocrinologist: This is a medical doctor with advanced training in the study of hormones and the endocrine system. This is the doctor who is an expert on diabetes who can help you manage your disease. Some endocrinologists further specialize in the treatment of diabetes (rather than other endocrine problems); these doctors are sometimes referred to as diabetologists.

- Diabetes nurse educator: Typically, the physician prescribes the initial treatment and insulin protocol, and a diabetes nurse educator works with the patient to provide follow-up care and to answer the many questions patients inevitably have about living with diabetes. The nurse educator often helps people with diabetes change their insulin plan as insulin demands change over time.

- Dietitian: A dietitian can help you learn to make wise food choices and to count carbohydrates so that you know how much insulin to take. Registered dietitians have been certified by the American Dietetic Association. A dietitian can help you come up with a customized meal plan that takes into account your personal preferences as well as your overall health.

- Ophthalmologist: An ophthalmologist is a medical doctor with expertise in managing diseases of the eye. It is essential that every person with diabetes has regular eye exams so that any diabetes-related eye diseases can be controlled at the earliest stages.

- Podiatrist and foot specialist: People with diabetes need to take special care of their feet, and podiatrists, orthopedists, and physical therapists can help. Podiatrists can assist with routine care, such as toenail trimming, as well as specialized care of structural problems with the feet.

Working with Your Team

It is essential that you develop a good working relationship with the experts on your health-care team. You should expect to feel comfortable and communicate well with each of your doctors. If a doctor isn't a good match for you, switch to someone else with whom you feel more comfortable.

When you go to the doctor, have your records updated and clearly recorded. If you have any questions or concerns, you might want to jot them down so you can be sure to get answers during the visit. Also, feel free to take notes at your appointments to clarify what changes you may need to make in your treatment.

Be sure you know how to contact your doctors in case of emergency. Every doctor has a particular way of handling after-hours emergencies. You'll want to keep the primary care doctor informed of various changes in your treatment, so find out how you should share information among your specialists.

When you leave the doctor's office, you may feel overwhelmed with the demands of carrying out all that you have been told. You may want to join a support group so that you can talk to other people who have more experience with diabetes. The American Diabetes Association and many hospital and universities sponsor support groups for diabetics. Many of the organizations founded to help people living with diabetes are listed in the section titled Organizations and Web Sites of Interest on page 276.

Diabetes Checkup

As a diabetic, you will need to have a number of tests performed regularly to assess your health and to determine if you need to be more vigilant in your self-care. You should have the following tests done regularly:

- Dilated eye exam: Once a year you should see an ophthalmologist for a complete eye exam, even if your vision seems fine. Be sure to let the doctor know you have diabetes.

- A1c test: Once every three months you should have this blood test done to assess how well you have managed your diabetes over the period. Talk to your doctor about setting a goal for your A1c results.

- Foot exam: You should check your feet for signs of neuropathy every day when you shower. Your doctor should check your feet at every regular appointment.

- Dental exam: Visit your dentist every six months. Be sure to mention that you have diabetes.

- Microalbumin test: Your doctor should test for protein in your urine at least once a year, more often if you have signs of kidney disease. This test is used to assess how well your kidneys are functioning.

- Blood pressure check: Your doctor should check your blood pressure at every appointment since many people with diabetes develop high blood pressure. As a general rule, you want your blood pressure to be under 140/80.

- Cholesterol test: Every year your doctor should test your cholesterol. People with diabetes are at increased risk of heart disease, so it is particularly important to avoid elevated cholesterol. Strive to keep your LDL (bad) cholesterol less than 100 mg/dl, your HDL (good) cholesterol 40 mg/dl for men or 50 mg/dl for women. Both men and women should keep their triglycerides below 150 mg/dl.

- Flu shot: People with diabetes and their family members should have flu shots every year, preferably in October or November. (Flu shots are not recommended for people with allergies to eggs.)

As you can imagine, working with these specialists and tending to your health care can be a daunting—and sometimes overwhelming—task. Many people with diabetes become frustrated with the chronic nature of the disease over time, and some experience depression as a result. The following chapter discusses depression and the emotional challenges faced by people living with diabetes.

CHAPTER 24
FACING DEPRESSION AND EMOTIONAL CHALLENGES

About six weeks after my six-year-old daughter was diagnosed with type 1 diabetes, I had to wake her up at 2 A.M. to test her blood sugar level. She was tired, irritable, and not the least bit interested in cooperating with me. She had been an extraordinarily good sport about her diagnosis—never complaining about finger pricks or injections—so I was worried that her sudden irrational behavior was caused by a potentially dangerous low.

I wasn't willing to forcibly test her as long as she was coherent, and she wasn't willing to accept my comfort until she had raged for every bit of 45 minutes. She cried; I cried. As suddenly as it started, her torment stopped. She looked up at me and said, "I guess I should test." Her blood sugar was a perfectly acceptable 145.

I held her for a few minutes and asked what she was feeling. At first, she shrugged. When I told her it was okay to be mad and frustrated, she said, "Mom, sometimes my bravery runs out."

I knew just how she felt. Since word of the diagnosis, we had each been trying to be brave for the other. I told her that I didn't want her to feel she needed to be brave all of the time. I invited her to share her feelings of loss and disappointment and fear and anger. Since then, she has remained heroic and brave, most of the time. And when she gets cranky (especially when we have to test at night), I try to reassure her that she's doing a great job.

Diabetes is an exhausting disease that will inevitably take its toll on even the most good-natured among us. As I learned from my daughter, it's okay to get mad at the disease and let off a little steam every once in a while. I try to encourage her to identify and express her complex and ever-changing feelings about living with diabetes, so that we can work together to make sense of the many emotional challenges she must face as a child with a lifelong chronic medical condition.

Dealing with Depression

Many people with diabetes experience depression. In fact, a 2003 study by the Centers for Disease Control showed that people with diabetes may be twice as likely as people without the disease to suffer from clinical depression. People who experience complications or have difficulty maintaining stable blood sugar levels may feel out of control and frustrated, which can contribute to feelings of depression. When you feel depressed, it can make it even more difficult to find the energy to work on good self-care. Depression should be taken seriously as a mental health complication of diabetes and treated with the respect it deserves.

Depression isn't the same thing as feeling sad now and then. Everyone feels down sometimes. Depression involves more intense feelings of hopelessness and despair. Depression affects thoughts, feelings, and the ability to do things everyday. Anyone, at any age, can have depression, but the risk is higher in people with a chronic condition, such as diabetes.

Depression can be effectively treated with antidepressant medicine, psychotherapy (counseling or talk therapy), or a combination of both. Getting treatment can help people better manage their diabetes and improve their quality of life.

Classic symptoms of depression include:

• Sad, anxious, or empty mood

• Feelings of hopelessness and pessimism

• Feelings of guilt, worthlessness, and helplessness

• Loss of interest or pleasure in activities that used to bring you joy

• Decrease in energy or feeling fatigued

• Difficulty concentrating, remembering, making decisions

• Changes in sleep patterns—either difficulty sleeping or sleeping too much

• Changes in appetite resulting in either significant weight loss or gain

• Restlessness or irritability

- Thoughts of death or suicide if depression is severe

If you experience three or more of the symptoms listed above or if you have one or two symptoms that last for two weeks or more, seek professional help. Talk to your doctor about your feelings; in some cases, a medical problem may be the cause of your emotional upset. For example, thyroid problems and certain medications can cause symptoms of depression. If your doctor cannot detect a physical cause for your depression, ask for a referral to a mental health expert. Look for a therapist familiar with the problems associated with diabetes, if possible.

Many people with depression attempt to "self-medicate" and develop problems with alcohol or other drugs. Substance abuse problems can make it virtually

---

CAN DEPRESSION CAUSE TYPE 2 DIABETES?

Chronic depression appears to increase the risk of developing type 2 diabetes, according to the April 23, 2007, edition of the *Archives of Internal Medicine*. The study of nearly 4,700 people over age 65 found an increased incidence of diabetes among people with depression, independent of other risk factors. The researchers theorize that the stress hormone cortisol, which is high during periods of stress and depression, may interfere with insulin sensitivity.

impossible to achieve good control of diabetes. Professional help will go a long way toward getting better and staying better.

Diabetes Doesn't Take a Vacation

At this point, diabetes can be controlled but not cured. If you have diabetes, you must deal with it every day of your life—on weekends, on your birthday, on holidays, on days you feel exhausted, on days you want to go to the beach, and on days you don't feel well (in fact, you need to take special care of your diabetes on days you don't feel well). Diabetes never takes a vacation, and that can take a real toll on your state of mind.

Being diagnosed with diabetes is a major life stress. It will require a new way of thinking about your health and your lifestyle choices. Many mental health experts believe that a newly diagnosed diabetic must go through the classic stages of mourning—denial, anger, depression, and acceptance.

Denial: Many people refuse to accept the diagnosis of diabetes, sometimes refusing to acknowledge the condition to their family or friends. The "honeymoon period," during which type 1 diabetics may need little or even no insulin, makes it especially easy for some people to deny the condition. Denial can foster feelings of loneliness and self-blame, which make it more difficult to move toward acceptance. It's hard to build a network of support if you deny the problem. In addition, if you keep your diabetes a secret, you could also have a diabetes-related emergency and no one would know what was happening, so they could not offer appropriate assistance.

Anger: It's okay to be angry at the disease, but in the

long run it's essential that you work through the anger so that you can make peace with your condition. It can be easy to ask "Why me?" It can be easy to resent other people who don't have diabetes, especially when they are able to indulge in treats that you can't have. It's not fair that one person has diabetes—or any other disease—and another does not. But there isn't much any of us can do about it.

Depression: As mentioned earlier, being diagnosed with a chronic disease can be depressing. You have, in fact, had to accept a fundamental shift in lifestyle and health-care management. Living with diabetes requires frequent compromises and inevitable frustrations. Don't blame yourself for feeling down about it, but do seek help when you feel you're in over your head. You are not alone.

Acceptance: Some people make peace with their diabetes easily, while others struggle with acceptance time and again. My daughter had to grieve the loss of part of her childhood when she was diagnosed, and I fully expect that she will have to grieve again when she learns more about herself as an adolescent, a young adult, a mother, and countless other times throughout her life.

Diabetes will be your traveling companion on an emotional journey throughout your life. It won't be easy, but you can strive to walk peacefully with this companion, rather than resist and fight every step of the way. If you can't make sense of this disease on your own, seek professional help from others who can help you take care of yourself, body and mind.

Eating Disorders

When she was a freshman in college, Kristy allowed her diabetes routine to slip, and she put on some extra weight. Eager to lose the extra pounds, she used her type 1 diabetes to put her body into ketoacidosis. Rather than restricting her diet, she restricted her insulin intake, forcing her blood sugar into the 400s and 500s. Her body responded by spilling the excess sugar into her urine. She lost weight, but at an unknown cost to her overall health.

Insulin manipulation—sometimes referred to as diabulimia—has become a significant eating disorder among type 1 diabetics, especially women. (Eating disorders are about ten times more common in women than men.) According to some estimates, as many as half of all young type 1 diabetic women have used insulin manipulation to lose weight. This is an extremely dangerous—and potentially deadly—practice, and a clear sign of an eating disorder.

In addition to insulin manipulation, the other classic eating disorders are anorexia nervosa and bulimia nervosa. People with anorexia nervosa restrict the amount of food they eat, often consuming well below 1,000 calories a day.

At the same time, many anorexics resort to extreme exercise, often working out for many hours every day to burn calories. People with bulimia nervosa binge by eating large amounts of food in a short time, then purge the food by vomiting or taking laxatives and diuretics. Both conditions make it virtually impossible to have good control of your diabetes.

Talk to your doctor if you're concerned that you or a loved one may have an eating disorder. Common symptoms include:

- You weigh less than 85 percent of normal for your height, age, and frame.

- You have significant anxiety about gaining weight, even though you are underweight.

- You think you are fat when other people see you are thin.

- You exercise obsessively to lose weight, rather than to become fit.

- You have missed three or more menstrual cycles and are not pregnant.

- You deny that you have a weight problem.

- You binge at least twice a week for three months.

- You feel you've lost control of your eating.

- You use prunes, laxatives, diuretics, enemas, or other medications to lose weight.

- You force yourself to vomit after eating.

Eating disorders in any form can lead to medical emergencies. They increase the risk of diabetes complications because blood sugar levels go so high and remain out of control for long periods of time.

If you suspect you might have an eating disorder,

seek help, preferably from someone familiar with the special concerns of people with diabetes. Many people with eating disorders feel shame and an almost desperate need to control their eating, but the consequences of poor blood sugar control threaten both your long-term and short-term health.

How to Be Supportive

Diabetes will have an effect on every member of the family, so it's important to be sensitive to the way the family works with the person with diabetes.

- Don't try to be an enforcer. Whether you're dealing with a diabetic child, a spouse, a sibling, or even a parent, you should not see yourself as a member of the Diabetes Police. No one wants to feel that their behavior is being watched and criticized, especially by someone who does not have diabetes and cannot fully understand the frustrations and challenges of living with the disease. On occasion, you may need to look the other way and give the person with diabetes the opportunity to manage the disease on his own. Of course, you don't want to stand by and watch someone you love make poor health choices, but expression of support and concern are apt to be more effective than guilt and nagging.

- Keep tempting foods out of the house. The diabetic diet is a healthy diet for most people. Make it easy for yourself or for those you love to eat the right foods.

- Offer to exercise with your diabetic loved one.

- Consider joining a local support group or working with a diabetes organization, such as the American Diabetes Association or the Juvenile Diabetes Research Foundation. By talking with other families you can learn specific coping skills, in addition to gaining emotional support when you need it.

- Ask how the person with diabetes is feeling. It may be difficult for the family member with diabetes to open up about his feelings if you ignore the condition. It's okay to talk about the disease, and it's important to unload about your emotions every once in a while.

- Try not to complain if mealtimes are rushed or delayed because the person with diabetes needs to eat on a certain schedule.

- Be understanding if plans must be changed because the person with diabetes can't engage in an activity because of a blood sugar high or low.

- Don't talk about diabetes in public without permission from the person with diabetes. Some people want to keep their medical conditions private, and that should be respected.

- When the person with diabetes isn't experiencing good control or feels frustrated by the disease, make a special effort to be understanding.

- Forgive the diabetic's erratic or unpleasant behavior during blood sugar highs and lows.

In the long run, it is possible to use your diabetes to
develop an increased sense of self-awareness. Most diabetics who have reached the stage of acceptance are
coping well with the disease on a day-to-day basis. They
watch their diet and exercise habits and manage their
stress, taking excellent care of their overall health. Some
may, in fact, take better care of themselves than they did
before the diagnosis.

Part of good health care is knowing how to take care
of yourself on the days you don't feel your best.
Illness—even something as simple as a 24-hour bug that
causes diarrhea and vomiting—can cause serious problems for a person with diabetes. The following chapter
discusses sick days and how to plan for them.

CHAPTER 25
MAKING A SICK PLAN

Donna, a type 1 diabetic, came down with the flu while in law school. She felt miserable all weekend, and she couldn't get her blood sugar down much below 300. She skipped class on Monday and stayed in bed. When her roommate returned in the late afternoon, Donna was confused and shaky. Her roommate called for help and Donna ended up in the hospital until her symptoms passed and her blood sugar stabilized.

Sick days present special challenges to people with diabetes. When you're sick, your body makes hormones to combat the illness. Unfortunately, these hormones also raise your blood sugar and make insulin less effective at lowering glucose levels. This makes a simple illness potentially very serious to a person with diabetes.

The best way to manage sickness is to be ready for it. Create a sick day plan with your doctor so you won't need to second-guess your decisions when you don't feel well. The following four-step plan can form the backbone of your sick day plan, although the details should be established with your doctor.

In addition to when you suffer from colds and flu, you

may need to put your sick plan into action if you have an infection, a physical injury, dental problems, an emotional crisis, or if you're recovering from surgery. Under these physically stressful circumstances, your diabetes will be more difficult to control and your blood sugars may run high.

Step 1: Keep Track of Your Numbers

You will need to continue taking insulin and other diabetes medication when you're sick, although you may need to adjust the dosage. If you have type 1 diabetes, check your blood sugar and ketone levels every four hours. If you have type 2 diabetes, check your blood sugar levels four times a day. If your blood sugar is more than 200, check for ketones.

By checking your numbers frequently, you can avoid developing ketoacidosis or hyperosmolar coma. (For more information on these complications, see Chapter 15.) Do not assume that you will feel the traditional symptoms of a high or low. Test and test often. Keep track of your results in your daily log book.

Step 2: Eat Right

Your diabetes goal when you're sick is the same as when you're not sick—you want to maintain stable blood sugar numbers. If you have a fairly minor illness, such as a cold, try to stick to the same foods you were eating before you became sick. If you need to modify your diet, try to consume the same number of carbohydrates in easier to digest foods such as soups and applesauce.

Check the sugar content of any over-the-counter medications you take, since many cough syrups and liquid medications contain lots of sugar. Some products are available in sugar-free varieties. You may need to adjust your medication to cover the additional sugar.

Nausea, vomiting, and diarrhea present additional challenges. You need to continue to take insulin and to consume an adequate number of carbohydrates, but you may need to switch to some foods that may be easier on the stomach than your traditional diet. The following foods each contain about 10 to 15 grams of carbohydrate:

- Frozen fruit pop or Popsicle
- ½ cup fruit juice
- ½ cup regular (not diet) soda
- 1 cup Gatorade
- 1 cup soup
- 1 cup milk
- 6 saltine crackers
- 3 graham crackers
- 1 slice dry toast
- ½ cup regular gelatin
- ½ cup ice cream
- ¼ cup sherbet

To avoid dehydration, you also want to drink at least 1 cup of water (or other sugar-free beverage) every hour you are awake. You may also drink bullion, broths, and clear soups, which contain sodium and electrolytes as well as water. Your urine should be pale yellow or clear. If you can't keep anything down—even clear liquids—be especially careful about monitoring your blood sugar.

Step 3: Take Your Medication

Take your normal dose of insulin or oral medication, even if you don't eat. If you take insulin, you may need some extra to correct for the high blood sugar during illness. If you take oral medication, you may need to take insulin to bring your blood sugar under control during the period you are sick. The details of your specific needs should be addressed by your doctor as part of your individualized sick plan.

Step 4: Ask for Help

Managing your diabetes is difficult under the best of circumstances, and it can be extraordinarily difficult when you're not well. Don't try to do it all on your own.

Whenever you are sick, you should let a friend or family member know so that someone will check on you regularly. If you are alone, it is possible to become confused and unable to care for yourself.

Diabetes complications can become dangerous quickly. You should discuss with your doctor in advance what warning signs should prompt you to call for advice. Be sure to maintain an up-to-date list of phone numbers for your doctor, which also includes emergency numbers so that you can call on weekends and holidays, if necessary. As a general rule, contact your doctor if:

- Your blood sugar is above 300.

- Your blood sugar is above 240 for two consecutive tests, even after taking extra insulin.

- Your urine ketone level is moderate to high.

- You feel unusually sleepy or fuzzy in your thinking.

- You vomit more than once.

- You experience diarrhea for a six-hour period.

- You have a high fever for more than 24 hours.

- You show signs of dehydration or ketoacidosis, such as difficulty breathing, fruity breath, or dry, cracked lips.

- You don't feel right and you aren't sure what to do to control your diabetes.

Before calling the doctor, check your current blood sugar, ketone level, and temperature. Your doctor may also want to know what you have eaten, what medication you have taken, and how much insulin or oral medication you have been taking. If you cannot reach your doctor, go to the emergency room, if you have persistent vomiting or diarrhea, difficulty breathing, or high ketone levels.

Even the healthiest among us succumb to illness now and then. By having a sick plan in place, you will know what to do to manage your diabetes when you're feeling under the weather.

Like sickness, travel can force you to change your diabetes self-care routine. It can be difficult to keep up with the changes in diet and exercise that can accompany out-of-town or overseas travel, but with advance planning you can control your diabetes and enjoy your vacation at the same time. The following chapter covers managing your diabetes while on the road.

CHAPTER 26
MANAGING TRAVEL

Gretchen carefully planned her family's trip to Disney World. She lined up the hotel, collected a medical letter from her doctor, packed twice as many syringes and alcohol wipes than she needed—then left home with the insulin still in her refrigerator. She realized her error after the plane had taken off. Fortunately, she also had packed prescription information from her doctor so she was able to replace the insulin at a local pharmacy when the plane landed.

Whether you're planning a day trip to the beach or a three-week European tour, you need to plan carefully to manage your diabetes when you're away from home. With some advance planning and a thorough understanding of how to change your diabetes routine, you can enjoy vacation and business travel without much additional stress.

Air Travel
The Transportation Security Administration (TSA), a division of the Department of Homeland Security, enforces a number of restrictions on travelers that can have

an impact on travel. Liquids and gels are restricted in carry-on bags, although they can be packed in luggage. (Airport X-ray machines do not hurt insulin.)

As a diabetic, it is essential that you keep in your carry-on luggage all necessary medical supplies, including a source of food to maintain appropriate blood sugar levels. The TSA has made an exception to the liquid-limit rule for medicines, including insulin. Insulin should be clearly labeled with the name of the traveler listed on the label. Also carry a letter from your doctor explaining the medical necessity of al the supplies you are carrying with you. To review the TSA rules, check the Web site www.dhs .gov/dhspublic.

When you arrive at the airport, let the security screener know that you have diabetes and are carrying medical supplies. You should be able to carry the following supplies:

- Insulin vials (with appropriate labeling)

- Syringes and insulin pens

- Lancets

- Blood sugar meter, test strips, meter testing solutions

- Alcohol swabs

- Insulin pump, batteries, tubing, and supplies

- Glucagon kit

• Urine ketone test strips

• Sharps disposal container

The screener may have you walk through the metal detector or visually inspect the insulin pump.

If you have trouble with a screener, you have the right to report problems to the TSA Consumer Response Center by calling 1-866-289-9673.

General Tips for Successful Travel

• Talk to your doctor about any changes in your insulin demands while traveling.

• Have your doctor write a letter explaining that you have diabetes and describing your medication program. Make several copies of the letter and carry one with you all the time. (It will be especially important if you have to go through customs.)

• Obtain prescriptions for all your medical supplies in case you need to replace them while you're away from home. Ask the doctor to write the prescription for the generic brand if you're traveling out of the country because most medications have different brand names throughout the world.

• You may be able to buy insulin and many blood glucose testing supplies without a prescription, but your insurance company may not cover your expenses.

- Test your blood sugar more often when traveling. Excitement and exercise can cause low blood sugars, so be aware and prepared.

- Always carry a source of sugar and testing supplies with you when you're exploring and out on the town.

- Pack about twice as many supplies as you think you might need while you're away. If possible, divide them into more than one suitcase or bag.

- Pack an extra glucose monitor—and don't forget extra batteries.

- Always wear a medical ID bracelet. (You should wear one at all times, anyway.)

- Be sure to maintain regular eating times.

- Carry insulin in an insulated container. As noted in Chapter 7, insulin should not become too hot or too cold. Keep insulin out of direct sunlight and don't leave it in a freezing car, even if it is in another container.

- Carry diabetic supplies in waterproof containers if you're going to a beach or to an amusement part with water rides.

- If you're going to a large amusement park, ask the guest relations office if you qualify for handicapped services. This may be able to help you qualify for early seating at restaurants if you need to eat at particular times.

Crossing Time Zones

If you're traveling across time zones, you will need to adjust your insulin dose. One method is to count the number of time zones you are crossing and dividing by 24. If you are going west, you increase your insulin by that much. If you are going east, you decrease it by that much.

Another approach is to simply add or drop one injection. If you're traveling from west to east, the day is shorter, so you should not take long-acting insulin and cover the blood sugar with short-acting insulin to avoid overlapping insulin. When you go from east to west, the day is longer, so don't eliminate the insulin but you may need to add an extra injection of short-acting insulin.

Another thing is to try to take insulin every four hours until your body has adjusted to the time change, then switch back to your normal routine.

If you're using an insulin pump, halfway through the flight, change the clock on the pump to indicate the time at your destination. This will change the basal rate of insulin. The bolus schedule should remain the same.

As you might imagine, frequent monitoring of your blood sugar level is the key to controlling your diabetes when you travel. The excitement of travel, as well as the changes in your diet and exercise routine, can create unexpected changes in your blood sugar levels. Bottom line: Test, test, test.

CHAPTER 27
DEALING WITH A DIABETIC CHILD AT SCHOOL

For me, the only thing more difficult than watching over my diabetic daughter day and night was letting her go to school for the first time after she was diagnosed with type 1 diabetes. I learned about her diabetes in the summer after kindergarten, and it took a real leap of faith for me to be able to let her go to school in the fall, confident that her teachers and the clinic aide at school would be able to handle any problems that would arise.

I was blessed to have a supportive and well-educated school nurse—and to attend a school already serving three other diabetic children, including two other first graders with type 1 diabetes. Still, for the first half of the school year, I visited the school daily to watch my daughter test her blood sugar and to help her count the carbs in her school lunch. I received regular calls from the nurse's aide every time my daughter went to the clinic to test when she felt high or low.

I realize that many other parents aren't nearly as fortunate. The bottom line is that your child has the right to be safe and well cared for at school and to participate in all school activities. That said, you may need to do your homework and become educated about your child's rights to ensure that your child has a successful experience at school.

Your Child's Rights

There are three basic laws that protect your child's rights: Section 504 of the Rehabilitation Act of 1973, the Individuals with Disabilities Education Act (IDEA), and the Americans with Disabilities Act (ADA) of 1990. They all basically say that your child has the right to go to school, take care of his or her diabetes at school, play a sport, join a club, and do the same activities kids without diabetes can do.

Section 504

A federal statute known as Section 504 of the Rehabilitation Act of 1973 protects all children with diabetes. Under the law, you are entitled to arrange for specific services for your child through written agreements known as Section 504 plans or Individualized Education Programs (IEPs). These plans create specific agreements on how your child will be granted the same access to educational opportunities as his or her non-diabetic peers. They can be particularly useful in allowing special accommodations for your child during standardized testing. Section 504 plans may be as detailed as you like, and they are customized to the particular needs of your child. While each plan is different, possible topics might include:

• Eating when and where necessary

• Going to the bathroom or drinking water as needed

- Participating in all extracurricular activities, including field trips

- Eating lunch at a specified time

- Missing school for medical visits and tests

- Timing of blood sugar monitoring and insulin injections, with personnel properly trained in the techniques

For more information on 504 plans visit the Children with Diabetes Web site at www.childrenwithdiabetes.com. The site provides sample plans at various grade levels that can be used as examples as you work out an individualized plan. You can also receive a school discrimination packet from the American Diabetes Association by visiting www.diabetes.org or calling 1-800-DIABETES.

Individuals with Disabilities Education Act (IDEA)

This law protects children who have a disability that affects their academic performance and ensures that all children receive a "free, appropriate public education." Your child may qualify for services, depending on how diabetes affects his or her ability to learn. Under IDEA, you also have the right to develop an Individualized Education Program with the school. This IEP is similar to the plan under the 504 Plan, but it includes specific measures to address your child's academic performance and special education needs.

Americans with Disabilities Act (ADA)

This law prevents schools from discriminating against people with diabetes and other disabilities. This law defines disability the same as in the 504 plan.

Doing Your Homework

Along with your child's rights come your responsibilities. It's up to you to make sure your child's teacher and the school nurse know everything they need to know about how to manage your child's diabetes at school. You need to work with your child's doctor to come up with detailed plans and you need to follow up every time your child's insulin demands change (which can be quite often).

Get to know the school nurse. You're going to end up having frequent contact with the school nurse or nurse's aide so that you can keep up with your child's health during school hours. Reach out to the nurse and try to establish a positive working relationship. Discuss your expectations about how you will communicate. Do you want the nurse to call you with your child's blood sugar level every day at lunch before administering insulin? Do you want to be informed every time your child visits the clinic because he or she feels high or low? Let the nurse or school administrators know what level of contact you need. Many times the school staff would appreciate your input on making medical decisions. After all, you know your child better than anyone else.

Teach your child's teacher how to recognize highs and lows. Your child's classroom teacher is the person most likely to notice if your child's behavior changes due to either blood sugar highs or lows. (My daughter gets verbose and loud when she's high and quiet, pale, and shaky when she's low.) By teaching the teacher about your child's individual warning signs, you can help your child identify possible blood sugar problems before they reach the crisis stage.

Create a supply closet for your child. At school your child will need testing supplies—a blood sugar meter, test strips, alcohol wipes, lancets—as well as snacks and juice or glucose tablets, and glucagon in case of emergencies. Typically these supplies are stored with the school nurse, although some schools may keep them in the classroom or the front office.

Prepare emergency kits. In addition to the main supply area, you will probably want to prepare emergency bags with snacks for other teachers your child will encounter during the day, such as the physical education teacher, art teacher, music teacher, librarian, and bus driver. Be sure the bags are clearly labeled. For my daughter, I prepared gallon-sized Ziploc bags with juice and Life Savers inside. A sheet of paper taped to the bag contains the following information:

- TYPE 1 DIABETIC

- Name

- Recent school photo

- Classroom teacher

- Warning signs of LOW blood sugar

- In case of emergency, dial 9-1-1.

• List of contact numbers for me, my husband, the doctor, and the hospital.

With these bags on hand throughout the school and on her school bus, my daughter should have access to quick carbohydrates if she ever needs them during an emergency.

Share what you know about diabetes. Set up a meeting with the school nurse, your child's teachers, and perhaps the principal to discuss the best way to care for your child at school. You should explain the basics of diabetes and how the disease may affect your child at school.

You can get information about diabetes and how it's treated from the American Diabetes Association, by calling 800-DIABETES. Ask for the free brochure, "Children with Diabetes: Information for Teachers and Child Care Providers." You can obtain a copy of a publication called "Helping the Student with Diabetes Succeed: A Guide for School Personnel" from the Juvenile Diabetes Research Foundation International at www.jdrf.org.

Offer to do a class presentation. You may want to make a brief presentation to your child's class to explain about diabetes. Most kids are inherently interested in how the body works and will respond well to the information if you present it in a positive way. When I spoke to my daughter's first-grade class, I showed them an insulin syringe and told the kids my daughter had to have shots four times a day. They developed a sincere (and well deserved) respect for my daughter's bravery, and they listened when I told them that while no one wants to be stuck like a pincushion every day, it really is quite remarkable that we have the medical knowledge to treat diabetes. If you're positive, the kids will be positive, too.

I also asked the kids if they could help my daughter by watching out for signs that she is too low. By teaching them about diabetes, they can become part of an extended network of caregivers who help care for my daughter when I am not there. Of course, talk to your child before you schedule a presentation. Some kids may not want the extra attention of a show-and-tell type session.

Food at School

School-age children love to celebrate their birthdays, and part of the excitement often involves cupcakes and other treats at school. With 25 or 30 kids in a class, that adds up to a lot of cupcakes in the classroom. Since portion sizes vary from one cupcake to another—and an extra glob of frosting can add quite a few carbs—you'll probably need to look at any treat yourself before your child eats it so that you can know how much extra insulin is necessary.

I encouraged my daughter to bring home any treats that she wanted to eat so that we could work them into her meal plan later in the day or the following day. She has been a good sport about wrapping them in paper towels and bringing them home untouched (so far, at least). Some children might have trouble resisting the temptation to taste the frosting or sneak a bite, but I think she liked carrying the treats with her on the bus.

There are a number of ways you might handle the birthday challenge:

- You could ask your child to skip the treat and not worry about it. (Ultimately, this is the approach we had to go to once my daughter was diagnosed with celiac disease on top of diabetes, meaning she couldn't eat the cupcake even if she brought it home.)

• You could stock the classroom with a box of low-carbohydrate snacks that your child could have only at birthday time.

• You could allow your child to eat part or all of the treat and then do a correction bolus at home.

Some kids struggle with the special treat issue, while others take it in stride. You'll also have to work out a plan for dealing with Halloween and other holiday treats. (I let my daughter eat a few things on Halloween and bolus for them, then snack on small treats for a couple of days. We freeze a little bit of candy and donate the rest to a local homeless shelter.)

When You Have Trouble at School

While most parents have very positive relationships with their teachers and schools, on occasion some parents encounter resistance from teachers and school officials about the care of their diabetic children. For example, some teachers have refused to let children have snacks in the classroom or attend field trips unless a parent comes along. Others have not allowed children with diabetes to participate in sports or after-school activities because the nurse is not available after hours to handle any diabetes-related problems. These restrictions are, in fact, illegal. Your child has the right to participate in all school activities, including after-school programs and sports.

While it makes sense to make every attempt to resolve any conflicts the easiest way possible, at times legal action is required. If your child is denied access to a school program, contact the American Diabetes Association or Juvenile Diabetes Research Foundation International (listed at the back of the book) for advice on how to persuade the school to allow your child to participate in all activities.

An adult with diabetes faces many of the same challenges in the workplace that a child faces at school. Discrimination is wrong at school, and it is wrong at work. The following chapter discusses your rights and responsibilities as an employee with diabetes in the workplace.

CHAPTER 28
WORKING

A waiter at a restaurant asked his manager where he could dispose of the syringes he used to inject insulin. A secretary at an insurance agency sucked on a piece of hard candy at her desk when she felt her blood sugar was dropping too low. A sales clerk in a department store needed to leave her post before her regular break in order to test her blood sugar when she thought she was experiencing hypoglycemia.

In each case, the employees lost their jobs once their employers learned about their diabetes.

Even though it is unfair, some employers discriminate against people with diabetes in the workplace. In most situations, this isn't due to malice, but rather to fear of high health-care costs or ignorance about the disease. Fortunately, you have specific legal rights as a worker with diabetes, and you can take specific steps to make sure you are treated fairly at work.

Your Rights
The Americans with Disabilities Act (ADA) and Title V of the Rehabilitation Act of 1973 offer protection to you

as a worker with diabetes. In a nutshell, these laws state that employers can't discriminate on the basis of a handicap as long as the person can perform the job with reasonable accommodations made by the employer. Under the law, diabetes is considered a covered handicap. Your diabetes cannot be used to unfairly limit your employment or advancement within a job, unless the disease prevents you from doing a specific job. If you are fired because of your diabetes, your employer must be able to prove in court that your medical condition interfered with your job performance.

In addition, your employer must provide "reasonable accommodations" for your diabetes. Alas, the law does not define the word "reasonable," and since every job is different, there is not a definition of "reasonable" that pertains to every situation. Some employers may be willing to provide regular breaks for blood sugar testing, snacks, and limited night hours, while another may not. In many cases, such disputes about what is reasonable end up going to court.

The federal laws do not protect every employee in every situation. The Americans with Disabilities Act applies to private employers, labor unions, and employment agencies with 15 or more employees and to state and local governments. The Rehabilitation Act of 1973 generally covers employees who work for the executive branch of the federal government or for an employer that receives federal money. The Congressional Accountability Act covers employees of Congress and most legislative branch agencies. In other words, employees of small companies may not be covered by any of these federal regulations.

In addition to federal law, all states have their own antidiscrimination statutes. Some of these protections are stronger than the federal laws.

Interviewing for a Job

You have the right to keep your diabetes a private matter during the initial job interview process. A potential employer has the right to ask you if you have a medical condition that could interfere with your ability to do the job—but not to ask specifically if you have diabetes (unless diabetes would interfere with your ability to do the job). The employer is expressly not allowed to give you a list of diseases and ask you have any of them.

If an interviewer asks about your health status, don't lie, but don't give any more information than you are required to by law. You might say, "I do not have any medical problems that would interfere with my ability to do this job"—as long as that is, in fact, true. Don't create an adversarial relationship (you don't have the job yet), so try to focus on all the reasons you are the right person for the job.

In many cases, your diabetes will be discovered during a physical exam prior to hiring. At this point, the prospective employer is seriously interested in hiring you and if you lose the position because of the diabetes, you have stronger legal footing to claim that you have been discriminated against. Be honest, but be cautious about sharing your medical history.

Some employers worry about hiring people with diabetes (and other illnesses or handicaps) because of their concern about high health insurance premiums. No doubt about it, diabetes is an expensive disease to treat, but anxiety about possible insurance claims is not a reasonable reason to avoid hiring—or to fire—a qualified employee.

Working with Diabetes

Okay, once you get the job, what will it be like to manage your diabetes while managing the workload? It de-

---

DIABETICS NEED NOT APPLY

There are a few jobs that are not well suited for people with diabetes. While there are a few exceptions, the Federal Bureau of Investigation has a policy of allowing diabetics taking insulin to become special agents. People with diabetes cannot enlist in the U.S. military, and many who develop the disease after enlisting must leave the service. Federal regulations prohibit diabetics who take insulin from interstate trucking, and many states also restrict access to intrastate trucking and bus driving jobs.

Additional regulations limit people who take insulin from becoming pilots and heavy machine operators; the rules on hiring police officers vary, but many do not allow diabetics taking insulin to join the force. In each case, the limitation on employment is intended to protect the diabetic employee, as well as those who could be harmed if the person experienced a diabetic crisis.

---

pends on the job and working conditions—as well as how you choose to handle your diabetes. People have succeeded in almost every job imaginable, from professional athlete to rock star to business executive, but only you know whether you're in control of your diabetes or if it's in control of you.

You also need to assess how you physically respond to a job. You may find dealing with a particular boss very stressful, which can interfere with blood sugar control. In time, you may be able to manage the stress or find a way to adjust your insulin, but you may also find it's easier to find another job with a better boss or a lower stress level. Some people can handle long hours, irregular hours, or shift work and still maintain good blood sugar numbers, while other people find that the disruption in their daily routines undermines their ability to control their diabetes. In other words, your situation is unique, and it's up to you to decide whether you are able to do a good job at work and do a good job taking care of yourself at the same time.

No matter where you work, you want to avoid having insulin reactions at work. It's impossible to predict every incidence, but you can go a long way toward minimizing your risk if you test often and identify patterns in your blood sugar levels. Keep juice, hard candies, or other sources of sugar with you at all times. Let your coworkers know how they can help you if you experience a low while on the job.

If You Experience Discrimination

If you believe you are a victim of discrimination in the workforce, contact the American Diabetes Association, your union, or an attorney for help. Keep copies of all correspondence from your employer, including e-mails and a log of phone conversations.

People who work for a private company or state or local government should file a charge with either the Equal Employment Opportunity Commission (EEOC) or the state antidiscrimination agency. You must act quickly because the time limits on filing a claim tend to be fairly limited. Since the exact regulations vary from state to state and case to case, it's best to begin the process by gathering information about the antidiscrimination laws that apply to you.

Once hired, you have the responsibility to be an excellent employee and to take the best care of your diabetes that you possibly can. You need to continue to practice good self-care and to manage your sick days and medical appointments in a way that minimizes the impact on your job performance.

Your diabetes does not have to limit your employment or performance at the vast majority of jobs. Your diabetes does not need to limit you in the workforce any more than it should limit you in other areas of your life.

CHAPTER 29
TAKING PART IN A CLINICAL TRIAL

In 1922, researchers Frederick Banting and Charles Best performed an important clinical trial: They injected pancreatic extracts into a 14-year-old boy who was dying of diabetes. The boy's blood sugar levels dropped to a safe level, and he lived to age 27. This was the first human test of the newly discovered hormone known as insulin.

Today, people with diabetes can choose from a number of insulin formulations, and those with type 2 diabetes have an expanding range of choices in oral medications. New medications and treatments—such as islet transplantation or stem-cell therapy—are in development and used in clinical trials.

Clinical trials typically involve experimental procedures, medications, or combinations of procedures. Some people join trials because they want to further medical science, while others feel that their lives may be enhanced by the possibility of a new treatment.

Clinical trials are essential for the advancement of diabetes treatment. Trials are the primary way medical researchers test potential drugs and treatments to determine their safety and effectiveness.

Most people have a preconceived bias toward trials, either imagining study participants being used as human guinea pigs to test dangerous, unapproved drugs, or envisioning test subjects as having the inside track on acquiring miracle medicines years before they are available to the public.

Frankly, trials are far more mundane than either extreme. While not free of all risk, clinical trials are typically quite safe. Checks and balances are built into the research process, including oversight boards to monitor the trials and to protect the health of the participants.

Clinical trials don't manufacture miracle cures, unfortunately. Diabetes is a difficult disease to treat, and progress is often incremental. The process can be quite tedious. Clinical trials progress slowly from one stage to the next, usually starting with a theory and laboratory testing, then gradually moving into the realm of human research. In addition, it must be noted that many clinical trials simply refine existing treatment protocols, without exploring wholly new approaches to treatment.

What Is a Clinical Trial?

Clinical trials are research studies in which people help doctors find ways to improve medical care. Each study poses a specific scientific question. Clinical trials can be sponsored by government agencies, cooperative research groups, private drug and biotechnology companies, or even individual doctors. They may be conducted in university hospitals, medical centers, community hospitals, or private doctors' offices. A study may take place at one or two locations or in dozens of centers nationwide, with results being submitted to a central location.

Sometimes doctors recommend patients for clinical trials, other times patients learn about various studies in progress and ask the doctor for more information. Whether the subject is raised by you or your doctor, it is essential that you openly discuss the topic with your health-care provider to determine whether participating in a trial is right for you.

Pros and Cons of Participating in a Trial

Clinical trials by definition involve testing on human subjects. While every precaution is taken to prevent harmful side effects, patients may face some risk. Experts review and try to predict side effects, but it is impossible for researchers to identify every possible consequence of a new medicine or treatment. In fact, initial or Phase 1 trials have as their goal detecting the side effects and tolerability of a new drug or treatment as the dose is escalated. Before agreeing to participate in a trial, a patient should be aware of all the possible risks and benefits that could occur by taking part in the research.

Most patients who participate in clinical trials receive excellent individualized medical care and benefit from taking part in a trial, whether or not the agent being tested in the trial is proven to be effective. Patients in trials often receive ongoing treatment from three or four physicians as well as research nurses. In many studies, there are mandated treatment schedules that require full physical exams every three or four weeks. This high standard of care makes it much more likely that any health problems will be detected and corrected, including even previously undiagnosed conditions.

In many cases, patients in clinical trials have access to new therapies or medications that they wouldn't have been able to obtain if they weren't in the trial. Don't participate in a trial expecting a miracle cure for your diabetes. No doctor can promise a particular outcome, although it is likely that your participation will further medical knowledge about the treatment of diabetes.

Of course, not every trial is suitable for every patient. To qualify for a study, you must meet specific eligibility criteria established before the trial begins. Even doctors involved in the trial can't make exceptions to these criteria and permit the participation of a specific patient.

Only you can make the decision about whether or not to participate in a clinical trial. Before you decide, you should learn as much as possible about diabetes and the trials available to you. Feel free to talk about this information with your doctor, family members, and friends to help you figure out whether or not a clinical trial is right for you.

In general, the potential benefits include:

- Your health care will be provided by physicians with expertise in diabetes.

- You may receive access to new medications and treatments before they are widely available.

- You will likely receive close monitoring of your health and any side effects of treatment.

- You will be able to take a more active role in your health care.

- You may be one of the first to benefit from a new treatment or medical device.

- You will be able to make a contribution to the existing knowledge about the treatment of diabetes.

The potential risks include:

- New drugs and treatments may have side effects or risks unknown to the doctors. Although it is rare, a new agent can have unexpected, life-threatening consequences.

- New drugs and procedures may be ineffective or unsuccessful.

- Often, research trials involve more tests and office visits than routine care.

Before joining a trial, you will be asked to sign a detailed consent form. The consent form includes information about the study approach, the intervention given in the trial, the possible risks and benefits, and the tests you may have. It should provide all the information you need to decide if you would like to participate. It should include every detail, from how many times you will have to test your blood sugar daily to whether or not you will be reimbursed for parking expenses during office visits.

Signing a consent form does not obligate you to remain in a study if you want to drop out. The consent form is designed to protect you, not to compel you to participate if you are no longer interested.

Trials are divided into phases, depending on the type of question being asked. Phase I trials (also known as safety studies) evaluate how a new drug should be administered, how often it should be given, and what dose is safe. Phase II trials test the efficacy of drugs at a specific dose. Phase III trials compare the treatment to the current standard. Phase IV trials involve drugs that have been proven safe and effective. For ten years after approval, doctors must report to the FDA any unexpected adverse reactions to the drug or procedure.

Questions to Ask Before Joining a Trial

Before agreeing to participate in a clinical trial, you should have a frank discussion with your doctor. Consider taking a family member or friend along to the doctor's office for support and to help get all your questions answered.

Write down all your questions in advance, then write down the answers so that you can review them. If you feel more comfortable, consider bringing a tape recorder so that you can review the doctor's responses after the appointment, if necessary. Be sure to cover the following questions:

About the Study
- What is the primary purpose of the clinical trial? What is the specific treatment being evaluated, or in what way will this trial advance medical knowledge?

- Who is sponsoring the trial? The federal government? A private drug or biotechnology company?

- Why do researchers think the experimental approach may be effective?

- What is already known about the drug or treatment?

- What phase is the trial—I, II, III, or IV? (The earlier the phase, the more experimental the procedure or treatment.)

- Who has reviewed and approved the study?

- How are the study results and safety of participants being checked?

- How long will the study last?

- What will my responsibilities be if I participate?

- Will I be able to see my regular doctor? When do I see the study doctors?

- Where else is this study being performed?

Possible Risks and Benefits
- How will I benefit from my participation? (You may choose to participate in a study even if you will not personally benefit because it will advance medical knowledge about diabetes.)

- What are my possible short-term risks?

- What are my possible long-term risks?

- Do you see a reason this may not be the right trial for me?

- If the research is already under way, can you provide a synopsis of how the other participants have tolerated the treatment? (The research physician may not be allowed to know these results, however.)

- How many other people have received the drug or treatment in the trial or in previous trials? What are the experiences to date?

What to Expect
- What kinds of treatments or tests will I have during the trial?

- Where will I receive my medical care?

- Who will be in charge of my medical care?

- What is the track record of the primary investigator? How long has he or she been conducting trials?

- What procedures will I follow to report any problems or sudden changes during the study? Is the contact person available 24 hours a day by cell phone or pager?

Personal Concerns
• How could being in this study affect my daily life?

• Can I talk to other people in the study?

• How much time will it take for me to participate in this study?

Cost Concerns
• Will I have to pay for any part of the trial, such as tests or the study drug? If so, what will the charges be?

• What is my health insurance likely to cover?

• Who can help answer any questions from my insurance company or health plan?

• Will there be any travel or child care costs that I need to consider while I am in the trial?

Finding a Clinical Trial

If you want to participate in a clinical trial, start by discussing the matter with your doctor. You can also do research on your own to find out which studies are available. The Web site www.clinicaltrials.gov provides a registry of federally and privately supported clinical trials conducted in the United States and around the world. The Web site lists information about each trial's purpose, who may participate, location, and contact information. You can also obtain information from major diabetes Web sites.

Clinical trials provide a transition between the current state of medical care and future treatments for diabetes. The following chapter describes some of the breakthroughs in treatment that are on the horizon.

CHAPTER 30
LOOKING AHEAD: Hope for the Future

Every three days, I change the infusion set on my daughter's insulin pump and once or twice a week I change the electrode on the sensor of her continuous glucose monitor. She stabs her finger with a lancet at least six times a day. That's about 45 needle pokes a week, 196 a month, 2,352 a year. . . .

Understandably, she sometimes experiences diabetes fatigue, feeling weary of sticking herself with sharps. On these occasions, I try to allow her to complain and then comfort her with my sincere belief that the current treatments will only get better. Glucose monitoring will become less invasive and more reliable. Insulin pumps will become smaller and lighter. And, someday—sooner rather than later, I pray—there will be a cure for diabetes.

My belief is based on more than a mother's dream. Almost every day there are news stories about some promising breakthrough in the treatment of diabetes. Some of the most exciting areas of research include:

- Internal insulin pumps: These are insulin pumps that can be surgically implanted under the skin, usually in the abdomen. Every one to three months the pump's insulin reservoir must be refilled. Insulin is administered by a remote radio device (similar to a TV remote).

• Improved continuous glucose monitors: The current generation of continuous glucose monitors still requires the sensor to be inserted under the skin to test the interstitial fluid. Emerging technology could allow bloodless testing, so that a device could assess blood sugar levels without piercing the skin.

• Islet cell transplant: Researchers have met with mixed success at transplanting the insulin-producing beta cells of the pancreas. By transplanting the beta cells rather than the entire pancreas, the surgery can be much less invasive. Research in this area is ongoing.

• Biohybrid artificial pancreas: This approach attempts to prevent the immune system from attacking the transplanted islet cells by storing them in a protective membrane. The membrane allows the islet cells to be exposed to the blood glucose so that the cells can respond and secrete insulin, but the pores in the membrane are small enough to filter out the cells sent by the immune system to attack the cells as foreign bodies. The approach has been tried successfully in animal experiments.

- Type 1 diabetes vacdine: Since type 1 diabetes is caused by an autoimmune attack on the pancreas, researchers are attempting to stop the process before the cell destruction is complete. They are attempting to develop a vaccine against the viral triggers that seem to kick off the immune response that attacks the pancreas.

- Reversing the autoimmune response: Researchers have reportedly reversed type 1 diabetes in mice by injecting them with a substance targeted to kill only the white blood cells responsible for destroying the pancreas. With these harmful cells out of the way, the beta cells regenerate, effectively eliminating type 1 diabetes. Studies have not yet been performed on human subjects.

- Stem-cell transplants: Researchers have used adult stem cells as well as young patients' own cord blood to reverse or slow the progression of type 1 diabetes. A lot of promising research is underway. Research teams have shown that ordinary skin cells in mice can be reprogrammed to resemble embryonic stem cells. This approach could be used to create a new source of mature insulin-producing beta cells. Additional research is ongoing.

- Hormone treatment for type 2 diabetes: Researchers have found that the hormone osteocalcin helps the body control blood sugar. Animal studies have found that when mice with type 2 diabetes were injected with the hormone they lost fat, produced more insulin, and used insulin more effectively. No research has been done yet on humans.

The Outlook

Using the tools available today, you can avoid many—if not all—of the long-term complications of diabetes by keeping excellent control of your blood sugar. Testing your blood sugar is easier and less painful than ever before. Low-sugar foods are widely available, and food labeling is much more comprehensive than it ever has been.

In the past, most people with diabetes had average blood sugar levels in the 200s and 300s. The Diabetes Control and Complications Trial showed that most people were able to prevent and slow the rate of complications by maintaining blood sugar averages of about 155. If you've fallen short of your goals—either with diet, exercise, or testing—don't beat yourself up about it. Today you have a new chance to get it right.

Talk to your doctor about your overall goals, and ask for help if you're struggling to meet those goals. The organizations listed in the following section provide not only information about diabetes care but also links to community support and local groups that can help you manage your diabetes. You are not alone; millions of other people share your struggle to live well with diabetes.

ORGANIZATIONS AND WEB SITES OF INTEREST

AMERICAN DIABETES ASSOCIATION
www.diabetes.org
1701 North Beauregard Street
Alexandria, VA 22311
(800) DIABETES

CHILDREN WITH DIABETES
www.childrenwithdiabetes.com
685 E. Wiggins Street
Superior, CO 80027
(303) 475-4312

JOSLIN DIABETES CENTER
www.joslin.org
One Joslin Place
Boston, MA 02215
(617) 732-2400

**JUVENILE DIABETES RESEARCH FOUNDATION
INTERNATIONAL**
www.jdrf.org
120 Wall Street
New York, NY 10005-4001
(800) 533-CURE

**NATIONAL CENTER FOR CHRONIC DISEASE PREVENTION
AND HEALTH PROMOTION, CENTERS FOR DISEASE CONTROL
AND PREVENTION**
www.cdc.gov/diabetes
4770 Buford Highway NE
Mailstop K-10
Atlanta, GA 30341-3717
(800) CDC-INFO

NATIONAL DIABETES INFORMATION CLEARINGHOUSE
www.diabetes.niddk.nih.gov
1 Information Way
Bethesda, MD 20892-3560
(800) 860-8747

**NATIONAL INSTITUTE OF DIABETES AND DIGESTIVE
AND KIDNEY DISEASES**
www.niddk.nih.gov
Building 31, Room 9A06
31 Center Drive, MSC 2560
Bethesda, MD 20892-2560
(301) 496-3583